FIGHT CANCER

By Naila Abdulla Ph.D

Second Edition

Fight Cancer Copyright@2020 Dr. Naila Abdulla

All rights reserved. Printed in the United States of America and Canada. No part of this book may be used or reproduced in any manner whatsoever without written permission from the author, except in the case of brief quotations within critical articles or reviews.

Every effort has been made to ensure content accuracy in this book at press time. The author disclaims and owes no liability to any party due to its content depicting authentic journeys in the fight against cancer.

This book constitutes three narratives based on personal experiences and outcomes in their Fight with Cancer. The two contributing authors are survivors and reading their fight is both encouraging and inspirational. Although every reasonable attempt has been exercised at content accuracy, the writers assume no responsibility for errors or omissions in the information provided.

Please use this information as you see fit at your own risk. Your life and circumstances may not be suited to examples shared within these pages.

The author is not a medical doctor nor in the position of registered authority to give expert advice. All that is being shared is personal experiences and changes lives. How you choose to use the information in this book within your own life is completely your own responsibility and own risk.

Print ISBN- SECOND EDITION #9781989848241

Print ISBN #978-1-7775430-1-3

Ebook ISBN# 978-1-7775430-3-7

Dedication

To Sherbanu and Yasmin, beloved mum and sister for their valiant fight against cancer.

With Thanks and Appreciation

To the outstanding group of focused and disciplined stakeholders partnering for improved outcomes. They stretch from dogged determination and tireless spirit of my surgeon Dr. Austen, to oncologists Dr. Henning, Dr. Barbera,and Dr. Abdullah for their skills and capabilities, to attentive physician Dr. Shergill, to home health care workers, Vittoria, Frewoine and Jessica for their nurturing care. To Mansoor, Fayrid & Yasmine for your outpouring of concern and kindness, Nizar and Yasmin you were my angels with candles in the dark always there with a smile and genuine concern. Nilofar Karim, you were my oxygen when I was getting depleted during the most difficult time, thank you for your travels to assist me during my hardest moments. To the hundreds of partnership-powered volunteers and non-volunteers, relatives, friends and neighbours, thank you for your compassion, friendship and dedication in helping me through this journey with your food, prayers, fruits and flowers to cheer me in the deep recesses of oblivion. I pray you are rewarded a thousand fold for God knows who you are!

Table of Contents

Acknowledgments

This book is a product of talented individuals who have volunteered their time, patience and efforts to make it a reality. I had been approached by neighbours and Nilofar Karim (a friend) to give advice on how to navigate the emotional barriers of fighting cancer.

My deep appreciation to Nazim Karim, Parin Verjee, Roshan Hemani and Shiraz Kurji for editing this book and for their kind support, suggestions, promptness, patience and goodwill. I trust they will find this book worthy of their consistent interest and valid suggestions. If this book fails in any respects the responsibility is entirely mine.

My desire to create an awareness on the processes in cancer treatment and providing a narrative of my emotions and experiences, was possible through this book. I later discovered that writing was the easy part as I progressively got frustrated in grappling with other aspects like formatting, design and publishing. My perseverance came from Heather Andrews at Get You Visible and I appreciate her encouragement and support.

I have been fortunate to find a caring friend in Roshan Hemani, who with her characteristic gentleness and warmth agreed to share her journey in this book. Having the voice of another valiant fighter, Shamshad Asaria, provides for alternative perspectives of other individuals who bravely battled this disease to become survivors and lead quality lives.

Finally, I'd like to thank the general readers for their interest in reading this book for increased awareness. Awareness means educating yourself in understanding emotions, causes, risks, symptoms and medical processes in the treatment of breast cancer to help you and your caregivers make the right choices in coping and managing.

Knowledge is power!

Introduction

Long awaited dreams for an early retirement started with a move to dry weather in Chestermere, Alberta, where I renovated and furnished my home and revived a bucket list of repressed plans, dreams and goals. My love for travel prompted a process of finalizing winter travel plans when a routine annual mammogram and biopsy suddenly brought the realization that I had cancer. How was I supposed to feel? I reflected on my status as a single woman, the eternal optimist, invincible, making the most of life's challenges, but this was different. This devastating news had me muddle-headed and frightened that life would never be the same. For the first time I felt urgency in wanting to accomplish my 'to do' list and prayed for a magic wand to miraculously eliminate my sickness and make me cancer-free. Being alone does not free you of feelings of pain, anguish and anxiety but there is no one who genuinely cares to know of your obsessive ruminations repeatedly shifting to emotional concerns, fear, panic, daunting thoughts, and an out of control life with an unpredictable future.

When you hear the word "cancer" what do you think? What do you know? Why did you get it? Is cancer a disease, a death sentence, or fate? After having used the term "I have cancer" my life met with a life-altering experience. Feeling sorry for a cancer patient is normal as there is the mortality, their emotional roller coaster and things are a lot worse than they appear. Thus, this story is mostly a serious, insightful depiction of my journey with an **attempt at creating awareness**. Every cancer narrative hums inspiring tales of courage with anecdotal capture of pain, suffering, hope and fight because that is a true depiction of a cancer patient's life. How can any story be different? Many times, cancer is dreaded because it's a wake-up call for being on borrowed time. This narrative is no different as it is a true caption of my journey sharing some aspects you already know, but some you don't and at the very least it will create awareness on how to find strength and courage to cope with the unpredictability of your circumstance or that of your loved one. I encourage continued reading as it may inspire you to take charge of your well-being and become a warrior and not a victim.

Cancer affects people in all parts of the world and although it is an economic burden on individuals, families and societies, you must not allow these considerations to cloud your journey as you focus your fight with this disease. There are more than 200 types of cancers, usually named for the organs or tissues where the cancers form. I have breast cancer which is the most commonly occurring cancer in women and afflicts 22,000 Canadian women every year, with more than 5,000 dying each year from this disease. 'Statistics' would be a cold reference term as no afflicted individual or family can accept their loved one to be a number but sadly Canada represents over 1.1% of the 2 million global cases reported in 2018.

Many take comfort in silence and struggle with their disease, whilst I believe there is a need to create awareness. The number of new diagnosed cases in Canada is expected to rise by about 40 per cent in the next 15 years, in large part because Canadians are growing older. If no cure is found, then breast cancer will be a crowded market and will have to meet with adjusted treatments, programmes and services to match increasing demands. The Tom Baker Cancer Centre currently under construction is intended to supplement the current overcrowded Centre where the number of patients coming through the doors continues to stress patient care. Construction of the new facility is an indication of growing demand. The probability for the processes and delivery of treatments may change with the new Centre but it validates the need for creating an awareness to the growing number of predicted afflictions.

I have a cancer laden family history and now am facing my own diagnosis. To be a host to a sinister enemy for which there is no cure and which cunningly has taken residence and is gaining victory in my body is unnerving. I refute the notion of victim-blaming the cancer patient for poor dietary or lifestyle habits, as there is no research based evidence to support this. I have witnessed this disease afflicting family members who exercised, were organic food consumers, lived a consistently disciplined life and were free of any facile habits. I had harboured a lurking suspicion that genetic predisposition would rear its ugly head and was diligent in my different variations on diet, exercise, sleep, yoga, relaxation and practicing calmness. But being suspended between a suspicion and a possible reality was robbing me from living in the present and I abandoned cancer-phobia for living in the moment.

It has been two decades since my late sister's demise and the news of my predicament was shocking, surprising, and I wanted second, third, fourth and countless opinions until I could be told the information was inaccurate. I consoled myself that my family member experiences were dated and the time lapse had met with significant medical advances than just 'extracting (mastectomy) and burning (radiation)' making my flashbacks redundant. I pushed for open dialogue with the health care support team and shared my concerns for an aggressive genetic mutation, living alone in my home in Chestermere, new to the area and one hour drive from Tom Baker Cancer Centre.

My surgeon, Dr. Austen, was a good omen as he won my trust and confidence and I readily accepted his recommendations. Realizing the acumen of your surgeon, oncologist, geneticist, radiologist, as better informed professionals who understand your medical situation better than you ever will is of fundamental importance. You can ask questions to better acquaint your understanding of the type of cancer and your condition. I equally recognize that the conventional team administering the treatments are unfamiliar with holistic and nutrition therapies as their training is based on medicine. You can ask questions to better understand safe and effective therapies but understanding the vast and complex field of cutting edge ways to treat cancer for a lay person are herculean. My reading was focused on conventional medicine due to limited time and need for quick decisions. If time permits, I would encourage you to research integrative approaches as many patients speak of the merits of naturopathic therapy. We share different needs for information, some of us want to know every detail, while others prefer not to know anything leaving the decisions to the experts. I think of myself as the most important part of the team as it's my body so I like to think of myself as a partner and believe that the better I understand my disease and its treatments the more endurance I will cultivate to fight cancer. In reading this book you will be familiarized with the multiple processes in your journey.

We live in a changing world with highly unusual circumstances due to the Covid-19 pandemic that has postponed screening appointments due to my immune-compromised condition. Despite library closures with no research capabilities or access to books previously written, I have taken the opportunity to write this book. I empathise with those who are in the midst of treatment or in need of surgery during the Covid-19 pandemic. Having spent the past 14 months in isolation due to surgery and treatments, I trivialize the notion of another 6-8 months in self-isolation as I am adept and experienced to weather the storm of isolation.

Cancer knows no national boundaries, ethnicities, religion, gender or age. All journeys are dissimilar with many unknowns and no predictable outcomes. We have heard miraculous stories of advanced cases of cancer patients fighting the odds to become cancer free and living quality lives~ some people get lucky with odds any gambler would envy. You need to understand your risks of recurrence, treatment options, their pros and cons, including side effects. Just as no two people can be alike, breast cancer afflictions are varying and different. What I didn't know is that breast cancer does not kill but its metastatic spread to other parts of the body is the culprit. While there is some controversy over how to properly calculate the number of metastasized recurrences, the general consensus is roughly 20-30%. That means approximately 1 in 4 of breast cancer cases are likely candidates to lose the battle with this disease. I'm no gambler but I don't like these odds.

Oh how my life has changed! cancer, a morbid topic, has dominated my life in a pervasive manner from almost daily treatment visits to awareness classes, from frequent visits to the Tom Baker Cancer Library (when it was open) to better understand a vocabulary that expresses processes like biopsy, genetic testing, mapping, mastectomy, bilateral surgery, staging, treatment options, mutations, drugs, ports, baseline functions, ATM, TNBC, TNM, DNA, ER, PR, HER2 etc. The use of medical terminology also makes my narrative medicalise, for which I apologise. The medical professionals are patient, accommodating, empathetic and quick to explain terms and processes, when asked.

Unfortunately, my navigating nurse had met with an injury and was on sick leave, compelling me to research the medical terminology. Navigating medical terminology proved challenging and a raison d'etre for writing this book, as there are many others who find the research process overwhelming. Ultimately, it was good to research the medical terminology as I was quick to realize that it is vital for a cancer patient and their caregivers to not only understand the disease but be cognizant of lifestyle changes it will impose. Panic paralysis from the news must give way to a pragmatic approach to problem focused solutions as it will better prepare you to overcome the many challenges you will confront.

In writing this book, I have an eagerness to share that life is bigger than cancer and though you have no power over when a cure for cancer will be found you have the power to expand your life in your attitude, compassion, hope, etc. Everyone experiences complications of ill health, conflict, family separations, disruption in friend circles and support systems. No life is more challenging than another but the attitude with which one responds in coping and managing and using the lessons learnt as a blueprint for living. Having lost my mother at a young age, sent to England for higher education and living among strangers, I was quick to learn from experience.

I have been approached by friends and neighbours to give advice on how to navigate the emotional barriers of fighting cancer. At first I felt inadequate to provide advice to a newly diagnosed patient on a subject of which I had little knowledge, having barely survived months after my treatment and by no means cancer free. It dawned on me that I have more experience than a newly-diagnosed patient and my intent for helping others should begin now.

Contemplation to write met with counter arguments as humanitarian causes do not get as much ink or respect as profit making enterprises. Libraries have been closed with no resource material to supplement writing. Is it realistic to write with no profit objective? How would I cover the cost of creativity, printing and binding? Fortunately, volunteers have generously agreed to edit and provided ideas to self-publish to reduce actual cost of marketing and distribution. I have no intentions of making money from this book with all profits to be donated to the Tom Baker Cancer Centre or the Canadian Cancer Society. My voice depicts my journey, and I have invited Shamshad and a dear friend, Roshan Hemani, both of whom are survivors, to voice their journeys for a varied read. This book is a narrative of authentic experiences.

We are not professional writers but private persons publicly sharing our journeys in the hope that we can inspire your fight. Miracles happen and we wish one for you. The subject of cancer is serious and any attempt to lend humour to this narrative would not be appropriate. However, efforts to engage you are genuine and sincere and we hope this read will help demystify a complex medical subject by detailing occurrences that are not limited to medical but to physical and psychological aspects encompassing emotional, social and spiritual well-being. Nothing is without risk and you are not alone. I fervently hope that this reading not only resonates for you to find hope, strength and courage to fight your fight but for you to undertake tough and challenging decisions. If our stories inspire and help a handful, it's worth the effort and will have served our objective. I invite you to walk this misadventure as I share my feelings, treatments and journal of medical visits.

Annual Check-up and mammogram

I was 19 when my mother died from breast cancer and it was then that I realized that cancer does not show symptoms. She was in great health and seldom given to fever or any downtime because of flu or inflammation. Thus, annual check-ups became an essential part of my life. I wondered if my current disease could have had its roots in a condition I experienced when I was 35, healthy, prime of my life and at the peak of my career. I was required to undergo a physical exam at the Mayo clinic in Boston for an upgrade to an executive insurance package. Examination revealed a large fibroid on my uterus which they suspected to be cancerous. I was in excellent health, had no symptoms and insisted further tests be conducted at the Mount Sinai Hospital in Toronto, my home city.

Hysterectomy was performed revealing a fibroid the size of a cantaloupe and the surgeon deemed it essential to remove my fallopian tube and ovary on one side, luckily showing a benign tumour. My journey for do's and don'ts commenced with being forbidden any form of estrogen, plant based or topical application. This over a period of decades led to weakening of my bones. A family history of breast cancer, coupled with this surgery, made me a candidate for regular screening for BRCA1 and BRCA2 as my genetic mutation indicated a 72% risk of being diagnosed with breast cancer during my lifetime (compared to 12-13% for women overall). Surprisingly, I did not take the statistics to heart as I commenced a life-style of hard work, normal life and became a caring custodian for my health by observing screening every six months, despite scarring and hardening of skin tissue due to increased radiation from mammograms.

Mount Sinai hospital dropped me from their monitoring program when I turned 60, alleging I was no longer at risk due to low levels of hormones, estrogen and progesterone. Although, I was unable to commit to the practise of regular breast self-exams, my strict discipline for regular screening was on-going despite hardship with a process that's not only painful but uncomfortable. Having one's breasts compressed between two firm surfaces for 10 seconds per image, makes the time appear like an eternity. However, mammograms can identify small lumps and calcifications that cannot be felt by hand and I believed benefits could outweigh risks, so I apprehensively submitted to a total of four images during each visit. Every time I had a mammogram, my standard lament to the technician was to convey a message to the powers to introduce a gentler process for capturing black and white images of breast tissue.

My lay person advice is for you to be a good stakeholder in monitoring your body and health by informing your physician of any unusual occurrences and use their medical acumen for further investigation. Fortunately, I had not accepted Mount Sinai hospital's declaration of being risk free and continued annual mammograms (a week before my birthday) as I confirmed positive to every risk category detailed below:

- I am over 50 years of age and 82% of the cases of breast cancer occur in women over 50.
- I have a family history of breast cancer.
- I had shown mutations to BRCA1 and BRCA2 genes.

- I have had numerous previous breast biopsies for calcification of cells.
- I have never been pregnant.

I had no predicted symptoms but respected an annual check-up appointment with my physician, Dr. Shergill, who, after careful examination, declared me in good health and sent me for a mammogram as per usual. There was no reason to suspect otherwise, as I casually strolled in for a routine mammogram test. To my surprise, this mammogram resulted in a mammoth frenzy as the resident radiologist requested additional five images as I sat in the waiting room for repeated takes of each additional X-ray. I was not new to additional takes as past experiences have required these, but this time, upon the third take I grew uncomfortable. This chilling wait has been ingrained in the etches of my memory, as I was not only troubled at the discomfort and harrowing pain from the mammograms but the disconcerting thought of something sinister lurking in my body. The radiologist informed me that I had a mass close to my chest wall and sought an appointment for a biopsy two days later at the Foothills Medical Centre. Being an eternal optimist I was certain that this biopsy would be similar to the ones before.

Biopsy and Appointment with Surgeon

With my biopsy requisition in hand, I stood in front of the Women's Health Centre on a cold snowy November morning, hoping that the biopsy would reveal nothing worrisome. I consoled myself that this biopsy would be nothing more than a calcification of cells as per several past biopsies and aspirations. Having agreed to research testing, I was required to meet with a representative from The Alberta Cancer Research Biobank (ACRB) to provide a blood sample and execute permission for research prior to the centre conducting any further tests. ACRB is a provincial bio-banking program responsible for collecting biological samples which are used to support medical research for disease prevention.

My two hour biopsy procedure required a sample of cells from the tumour. My relaxed demeanour turned into stressful anxiety as I intuitively was full of foreboding despite the radiologist's gentle, caring and communicative search. With a sudden change in tone she informed me of the tumour cells being cancerous. I was informed that the lymph nodes appeared clean and samples of both had to be sent to the lab for confirmation. She referred me to the navigating nurse for Dr. Austen, Breast and Laparoscopic Surgery, for an appointment within two days of my biopsy. The speed for my appointment suggested urgency. Grappling with the worst news ever, I was in a state of shock with the reality of having cancer and my thoughts raced in all directions. I was surprisingly stoic but determined to understand the extent of my affliction.

To accept a stressful situation with calm and dignity, I assumed a 'stiff upper-lip' based on a tradition I learnt from the time I first left Kenya for England at age 18. My calm resolve turned to agitation as parking at Foothills hospital was impossible and I was increasingly late for an important appointment. Dr. Austen brought a change in my attitude as I asked rational questions to better prepare myself for the journey ahead. Dr. Austen was sympathetic, comforting, relaxed, and easy to talk to, with a 60 minute consultation passing swiftly as he not only answered my questions, but won my trust and confidence with his genuine caring attitude in preparing me as best he could. His genuine interest in me as a patient was important as he tried to better understand me, my lifestyle and my family history. He detailed an honest portrayal of challenges ahead and wondered if there were additional people to be present at future appointments.

I learnt that there are many types and subtypes of cancers and many variables that lead to different cancer characteristics. I had been diagnosed with invasive lobular carcinoma called an ataxia telangiectasia mutation (ATM), a genetic condition passed from my family. I learnt that ATM is a rare form of cancer having met with fewer cases presenting unpredictability of the efficacy of treatments, chemotherapy complications and their outcomes, with symptoms like essential tremors, lung disease and neurological decline. Invasive Lobular Carcinoma begins in the lining of the milk glands and provides for 5% of the total breast cancer cases. My chaotic world was changing rapidly not only in my emotions but my vocabulary, new people and faces, unfamiliar processes, new buildings and locations. I requested a genetic test and Dr. Austen booked me an urgent appointment with a medical geneticist at Alberta Children's Hospital. I left the surgeon's office with feelings of positivity, a surprising sense of strength and calm to map my future action chiding myself to be alright. I was emotionally calm and unaware of the reality of challenges ahead.

Every cancer patient's journey is different, some longer and harder than others. My awareness and preparation suggests that determining the stage of breast cancer is important (size and extent) as different stages have different risks of recurrence and treatments. Breast cancer cells may spread by travelling to lymph nodes in the armpit (axilla). I was informed that surgery would not only remove the tumour but lymph nodes if they needed to be removed. My consult with the surgeon had many unknowns and our discussion revolved around hypothetical situations as only surgery would unfold accurate details of my cancer.

Genetic Testing

Despite December being a short working month, given my biopsy results, I was fast-forwarded to consulting a geneticist. Before a genetic test was ordered, a consent form had to be signed, suggesting I understood the purpose of the test, its medical implications, risks and benefits, and privacy rights. I understood nothing but signed consent to proceed in giving a blood sample and a genetic chart detailing family breast cancer cases and outcomes. My blood sample was sent to a laboratory for genetic testing with results submitted to my surgeon and genetic counsellor. A genetic testing process can take three months but mine was expedited in five weeks despite the holiday period.

The genetic counsellor educated me on the many types of genetic tests and I underwent a genetic test for conformational diagnosis as a symptomatic individual. Despite having been diagnosed I underwent this testing for the benefit of biological relatives ~ genetic brothers, nephews, niece and relatives who could be susceptible. Sometimes cancer can appear to "run in families" as a single altered gene inherited from one parent can increase the chance of developing cancer. Most immediate to my mother and sister, who were both diagnosed with metastatic breast cancer at age 48, I have a history of maternal familial mutation through multiple generations with many cousins diagnosed at young ages suggesting a strong connection to hereditary link.

My unfair maternal family history laden with cancer stretches beyond my mother and sister to many aunts and cousins. Recent demise of my cousin Guli Adam, who was kind, caring, virtuous, wise, sincere, spiritual and smart. She was diagnosed with breast cancer with subsequent metastases into her blood stream. My cousin Shamim was in her early-thirties, very beautiful and had given birth to her daughter in Toronto, when she was informed of her breast cancer. She was a vegetarian, and looked after her well-being as her mother had suffered from this demonic disease. Prior to submitting to surgery she ensured milk was pumped for her little baby-girl and she stoically submitted to Divine Will as **what choice did she have?** Post-surgery recovery compromised her ability to provide for her young children and her worst fears were realized when her cancer spread to her brain and assumed victory in taking her life. My cousin Nabat, known for her stunning beauty, was in her early-thirties when diagnosed with cancer and underwent a bilateral in Nairobi, followed by chemotherapy and radiation in the early 1970's. **What choice did she have?** Her efforts to live on account of her three children aged 16, 13 and 7, failed as she succumbed to cancer in December of 1974. Two of her children living in Calgary have been diagnosed but luckily after varying treatments are free of cancer.

The geneticist ordered a 13-gene hereditary breast/ovarian cancer panel over a period of 4 week turnaround. My autosomal genetic test found a genetic variant for the benefit of my family awareness and for my medical team to better understand treatment options. My mother and sister ate organic and nutritious food and both still contracted cancer. My sister, also a beauty, multi-talented and with two masters' degrees, had a passion for life. She was an avid reader, worked as a librarian, loved art and designed the blue-print for building a house on a parcel of land near her home in North West Calgary. She had fought for every trial drug that allegedly could help her. Her treatments and records from 1995-1996 at Foothills hospital were not accessible. My fears of extreme pain, suffering, nausea and severe lymphedema stem from having been a care provider and observing her journey with the disease. The innumerable cancer cases in my family have occurred at a younger age. I feel blessed to have enjoyed two extra decades of a quality life. The good news is that I am single and have no children to worry about but I too have feelings, concerns and a bucket list, **but what choice do I have?**

Every trace of anxiety and stress evaporated as I idled my time in the Alberta Kids Hospital lobby, enjoying sparkling lights, glittering decorations, kids enjoying electronic gadgets, cookies and candy. The spirit of Christmas abounded as good cheer, love, understanding and volunteers' spreading goodwill to children who trustingly submitted themselves to the medical community for improved outcomes. Having popcorn, candy cane and cookies, I resolved to live each day to the fullest, partner with my medical team for treatments and **to share my experience and journey with others.**

Bilateral Surgery

My ovary, fallopian tube and uterus had been removed 33 years prior and now I was to lose my breasts to cancer. I pondered on the undue hardship and the impact of my failing health on my emotional wellbeing? Force of habit pushed me to stay positive and accept whatever I couldn't change. I believe that negativity is a failing to be avoided and surround myself with people who are positive and have a sense of humour. In fact, I was enveloped by a sense of gratitude at not having to contend with medical costs and being in a great country like Canada. The day prior to my breast cancer surgery, my cousin Nizar drove me to the Foothills Medical Centre Nuclear Medicine Department for a mapping procedure. This painful procedure locates and marks a group of important lymph nodes near the tumour. I was given two radioactive injections near the nipple and had to wait for three hours for the dye and radioactive substance to trace the pathway of the lymphatic system and identify the sentinel node.

As there was no need to remain at the hospital for the wait, I visited the Market Mall for lunch. Upon my return and in preparation for surgery, two images of my chest and armpit were taken. The night before surgery, I was prepared with my hospital overnight bag of recommended items and surprisingly succumbed to sleep as my head hit the pillow.

My brother Mansoor from Toronto, drove me to Rocky view General Hospital early morning on February 12. Being seated in a busy surgery waiting room, I observed a highly efficient process as electronic boards detailed the surgeon, his medical team and the name of the patient with estimated scheduled time for surgery. My wait was short as I was taken to a private room in the corner of a large area the size of a gymnasium court where hospital beds were curtained to allow privacy for short post-surgery recovery. I presume I was provided a private corner room due to an overnight stay.

Just prior to surgery I was wheeled on a stretcher to a waiting area in front of the operating theatre and provided with several warm blankets for comfort, this short wait was intense as it dawned on me that I was in for serious surgery. Suddenly, I was gripped by fear in anticipation of possible scenarios pertaining to the stage of my cancer and the unknown challenges of surgery. These concerns were short-lived as the anesthetic team introduced themselves, medicated me for a four-hour surgery and swiftly wheeled me into a very cold operating theatre. The nurses were prepared for lower back stenosis problems and propped my legs as they surrounded my feet and legs in soft cotton electronic covering for extra comfort. This attention to detail was extraordinary and I was grateful for a caring surgeon. It was a relief to see Dr. Austen's familiar face and with this source of warm comfort I commanded a warm, broad smile and muttered "please do not touch my lymph nodes" prior to succumbing to the power of anesthetic as I drifted into deep sleep.

Surgery is the most important first line of defense and the most effective in a fight against breast cancer. Dr. Austen had his work cut out for him in not only having to remove a sizeable tumor, perform double mastectomy but removing my sentinel lymph node and 16 lymph nodes in the armpit, a process referred to as an axillary lymph node dissection (ALND). He must have been surprised at the speed of my cancer growth. **My worst fears of cancer in my**

lymph nodes had met with reality. The side effects of ALND include pain, numbness and limited movement in the arm, shoulder, and probability of lymphedema. Lymph node extraction is also suggestive of the cancer having spread through the lymphatic system.

Dr. Austen informed me of having had to remove my cancer and lymph nodes when I first gained consciousness in the late afternoon and then again at 6.30 AM the following morning. He feared I may not have been lucid when he first informed me of removing some lymph nodes and was by my bed early morning to personally deliver outcomes of my surgery. His realization that I was single, living alone and new to the region brought a firm assurance of him being my family member, and available for any assistance or support I needed. My surgery outcomes had not been favorable as my tumour was 2 cm. large and 16 lymph nodes were extracted in the armpit, both considered significant. My worst fear had been realized in the predicament of the cancer having spread into my lymph nodes with an ability to travel through the lymphatic system to any tissue or organ. I learnt of the number of lymph nodes extracted from reading my pathology report as Dr. Austen opted not to tell me soon after surgery. The ramifications of this extraction are many and further reading will apprise you of its impact. Prior to undergoing surgery, I presumed that surgery is the most effective and probably the only major medical intervention in my fight against cancer. **Post-surgery I was informed that surgery is only the first step in many, making treatments crucial.**

Following surgery, I have no recollection of the nurses checking my vital signs, dressing and drains in the recovery room. I woke from the deep clenches of anesthesia in the late afternoon and recall my brother and Dr. Austen in my room. I was hungry and given soup, jelly, weak tea, and water, and was encouraged to walk. I felt like an alien walking connected to IV transfusion for fluid and pain killers. My overnight stay at the hospital met with the night nurse at 2AM showing me the procedure for draining blood from the three vials attached and to record the time and amount drained. Before my discharge the following day, I was provided with a drain and incision care instruction sheet, a prescription for pain medication, triage telephone numbers and a home care referral. For a post-surgery person, deep in shock and high on drugs that's a lot to absorb. The provincial health plan provides daily home care in the morning and evenings and my care worker promptly arrived as soon as I was home, to help with sponge bath, meal preps, exercises and massage which was necessary and a blessing. For a month after my surgery, Vittoria, a nurse arrived mid-day to change my bandages and check healing from the surgery.

Three drains were attached to my surgery area to help drain fluids and reduce the chance of swelling from fluid buildup. The drains were sutured and the initial dark red drainage lightened over time. My nervous anxiety and frantic calls to the nurse at little clots plugging the drain, met with instructions at clearing clots and through familiarity I became adept. For a period of 10 days the vials had to be emptied twice a day and after five days, once a day. My initial anxiety and discomfort at emptying the vials met with calm expertise within 48 hours and in 10 days the navigating nurse having returned from sick-leave removed the sutures. In retrospect, the processes which appeared daunting soon after surgery appeared doable and not so bad with practise.

From early detection to Metastasis

Now for a short lesson on genes to better understand why you have cancer. Genetic changes are sometimes called "drivers" of cancer and there are three main types of genes ~ proto-oncogenes, tumor suppressor genes and DNA repair genes. Proto-oncogenes are involved in normal cell growth and division. However, when these genes are altered in certain ways or are more active than normal, they may become cancer-causing genes (or oncogenes), allowing cells to grow and survive when they should not. Tumor suppressor genes are also involved in controlling cell growth and division but with certain alterations in tumor suppressor genes they may divide in an uncontrolled manner. DNA repair genes are involved in fixing damaged DNA but cells with mutations in these genes tend to develop additional mutations in other genes. Together, these mutations may cause the cells to become cancerous. As scientists have learned more about the molecular changes that lead to cancer, they have found that certain mutations commonly occur in many types of cancer. Because of this, cancers are sometimes characterized by the types of genetic alterations that are believed to be driving them, not just by where they develop in the body but how the cancer cells look under the microscope.

Breast tissue is supplied by blood vessels and lymph vessels. A lymphatic system circulates a clear fluid called lymph throughout the body. The lymph is filtered through lymph nodes which are small round structures filtering bacteria, viruses and cancer cells. The lymph nodes around the breast are grouped in four locations: the armpit, above and below the collar bone and inside the chest near the breastbone. Based on my late sister's lymphedema, I was fearful and apprehensive at the potential loss of armpit lymph nodes and shared my concern with Dr. Austen on one of my visits prior to surgery.

Cancer cells break away from where they first formed (primary cancer) and travel through the blood or lymph stream to form new tumors (metastatic tumors) which are the same as the primary one in other parts of the body. For example, breast cancer that spreads and forms a metastatic tumor in the lung is metastatic breast cancer, not lung cancer. In my case the spread most likely can occur through the lymph stream.

Under a microscope, metastatic cancer cells generally look the same as cells of the original cancer. The primary goal of treatments is to control the growth of cancer and to relieve symptoms caused by it which helps prolong lives for people with metastatic cancer. One can hope that a cure is found during the extension of life to make the journey and fight against cancer worthwhile. Metastatic tumors can cause severe damage to how the body functions, and most people who die of cancer die of metastatic disease. Lymph nodes being removed suggest cancer could have spread as lymph circulates throughout the body but there is no predictability as to where cancer cells could have traveled.

Understanding the stages of breast cancer based on its spread is **important** as it determines the treatment options. There are five stages of breast cancer, commencing with stage zero to four. Stage 4 means that it has spread to your organs and is the most advanced. Staging is determined by mammograms, ultrasound, biopsy, testing lymph nodes and surgical pathology report. Staging systems classify breast cancers according to the size of the tumour mass and whether it has spread to nearby tissues, to lymph nodes near the breast (armpit or axillary nodes), and to other tissues of the body (example. bones, liver, lungs or brain).

For statistical and research purposes cancer staging system called tumour node metastasis (TNM) is used and considers tumour size (T), lymph node involvement (N) and metastases (M). My large tumor appears to be triple negative breast cancer (ER negative/PR negative/Her2 negative) Triple negative suggests a high likelihood of spread and less likely to respond to treatments. I am stage 3C with cancer having extended outside lymph nodes into the fat tissue. Lymphangitic spread occurs when cancer travels through the lymphatic circulatory system and takes hold in different parts of the body.

The chapter of my journey of diagnosis, surgery had ended. Prior to surgery I believed myself to be a case of early detection. After surgery my realization has dramatically changed to being at high risk for recurrence and the question of if I will ever be cancer free? Despite a somber pathology report, I entered the ring for a vigorous fight for more than three minutes per round, hoping for a miracle:

- My ATM cancer is rare, has met with less attention, and is neurological.
- The tumour size is 2 cm. which is considered significant.
- My cancer is a triple negative, suggesting a high likelihood of spreading and less likely to respond to treatments.
- 16 Lymph nodes have been removed, which is considered significant.

- After treatment, I am at a high risk for recurrence.

The bad news is that my cancer is considered invasive and advanced with lymph nodes affected. The good news is that it hasn't yet spread to my organs. My cancer staging suggests a significant risk for local and systemic recurrence, in addition to an ATM which is rare, neurological and has met with limited attention. Despite this somber prognosis, I firmly believe the benefit ratio is in my favour today based on my current staging and therapy to be delivered. With this knowledge, I have opted for treatment anxiously awaiting the announcement for a cure soon.

Treatment

Prior to surgery I had resolved not to allow breast cancer to define me as I value my independence. I have been honest about my predicament and writing this book has been for the potentiality of benefiting another. These are tough times calling for tough decisions, and I will never know the right answer but I must give it my best shot. My initial concerns were now fast changing to forces I had not anticipated and chemotherapy treatment that I certainly did not want. I read about alternative therapies and spoke with two stage 1 and 2 patients who had adopted alternate approaches. Prior to my surgery I had toyed with the idea of being treatment free and fighting with healthy nutrition. However, after surgery and knowledge of my pathology report, I opted for a medical approach that would provide quick and aggressive medical intervention; in addition, I confess to not being a candidate for healthy nutrition as I am addicted to carbs, fries and crisps. My choice to pursue a medical path has no guarantees or known outcomes but I am set on this path and will follow it with diligence. At the onset, I had come to terms with my unfortunate circumstances and was determined to fight.

Cancer and normal cells multiply through cell multiplication repeatedly dividing. Cancer cells divide quickly, but so do some healthy cells. The goal of chemotherapy drugs is to kill the rapidly dividing cancer cells preventing them from spreading. As chemotherapy cannot differentiate between healthy and cancer cells the drugs damage rapidly dividing cells including normal cells. When healthy cells are attacked varying side-effects in each individual are created from the toxicity of the drug.

Different chemotherapy drugs damage the cancer cells in different ways, and in combining drugs the probability of treatment success is increased. Combining chemotherapy drugs is based on the ideology that the most effective way to kill cancer cells is to target many different processes in the cancer cell at the same time.

An appointment was scheduled with Dr. Jan-Williem Henning at the Holy Cross Centre on April 10. Through my fight with cancer little did I know that Dr. Henning would be the most consistent doctor to treat me through a series of chemotherapy treatments. Cancer treatment with its ominous reputation places the burden on the oncologist who works relentlessly for good outcomes. His job is probably the toughest in witnessing treatments failing and patients dying. Contingent upon my consent, treatment was to commence on April 25, 2019, and I understood from my oncologist that my cancer was 'tricky' and aggressive. An important decision to determine the best treatment option had me on the strongest chemotherapy drug currently available. I was agreeable to the most aggressive treatment suggested through systemic chemotherapy to be delivered at the outpatient Tom Baker Cancer Centre. Systemic therapies are drugs that spread throughout the body to treat cancer cells wherever they may be. My treatment was a cocktail of drugs infused to travel through the bloodstream, given in cycles giving the body time to recover before the onslaught of the next cycle. My oncologist used a protocol for 4 cycles of AC (Doxorubicin & Cyclophosphamide) every 21 days followed by 12 cycles of paclitaxel given weekly. My first chemotherapy session commenced on April 25 and systemic treatment ended on November 10. A great tip provided in the reading material states, "Feel secure and cared for in the treatment plan that has been created."

My lay-person learning surmised oncology to be delivered in protocols that are administered based on your cancer stage but every drug is a variation or combination of the three approaches outlined:

1. A chemical is tested and found to kill cancer cells while sparing most normal ones.
2. Discovering an active protein especially in cancer cells and targeting that protein with a drug.
3. Identifying some behaviour of a cancer cell that renders it uniquely sensitive to a chemical.

I view cancer cells as cunning as they have their own sustenance to be growing with in you.

1. Cancer cells co-opt neighbouring blood vessels to supply themselves with oxygen.
2. They enable their own movement through the body by hijacking genes that allow normal cells to move.
3. When some cancers metastasize in the bone for their survival, they imitate an accelerated form of osteoporosis.

Delivering chemotherapy at Tom Baker Cancer Centre was efficient and operated like clock-work. The first 4 cycles were administered for a period of three hours by two nurses who stayed with me as they monitored the flow of toxic drugs. Doxorubicin (Adriamycin) is one of the most powerful chemotherapy drugs ever invented. It can kill cancer cells at every point in their life cycle, and it's used to treat a wide variety of cancers. Unfortunately, the drug can also damage heart cells, and every six months my heart has to be monitored through echocardiograms. During chemotherapy infusion, a pump controlled the medicine flow from a bag through tubing that was attached to my IV. Side effects during this phase were strong and a close scrutiny was given during the first 4 cycles because of the toxicity of the drug. I mustered all my strength and determination for an indomitable fight against the side effects of chemotherapy, thinking this too shall pass. I reminded myself that though my body had weakened, my spirit was strong, I still had hope. The next phase was Paclitaxel, which was administered for two and half hours. A nurse seated in the centre of the chemo room across from each cubicle could be called by pressing a red button. Life is never free of challenges and this time veins for infusing chemo had become 'elusive,' causing me pain and difficulty for the nurses to find a good vein. Progressively it got harder on both the nurse and myself and this made me a candidate for another surgery for inserting a port. For every chemotherapy session I requested a window cubicle to enjoy natural light which promoted a sense of happiness and calmness. Exposure to natural sunlight allowed me the luxury of warmth from the golden rays allowing my mind and body to be relaxed. I enjoyed watching outdoor activity on Chinook days, and imagined myself enjoying lunch on the picnic benches. Intermittently drifting in and out of sleep, I was able to feel the warmth of sunshine streaming through my window lending extra comfort and happiness.

In my months of gruelling chemotherapy treatments, physical weakness and the overpowering need for sleep, I lost touch with the world around me. But once in my window cubicle in the treatment room, I lived joyously through virtual trips to flying with birds, gliding, and parasailing.   I indulged myself to the luxury of my wanderlust for travel and found myself cruising the Mediterranean, basking in the warmth of the sun and swimming in the South Seas to visualizing my journey through the islands of the Pacific Ocean and dancing the kalakeke. I recollected my past trips, yacht cruising off the coast of Vancouver, visiting northern Canada and land of midnight sun; eating lobster and crab on the Atlantic coast; being on a wildlife safari, travelling across the Himalayas; being on the Karakoram and visiting remote areas of Gilgit, Chitral and Hunza; visiting the Grand Canyon; enjoying the hula in Hawaii, the Great Wall of China and the Forbidden City; walking the grounds of Angkor Wat in Cambodia, the place of Gods; watching the whirling dervishes in Konya; visiting the pyramids and- cruising the Nile; shopping in Muscat bazaars; purchasing art in Udaipur; strolling the charbaghs of Taj Mahal admiring the intricate dome and minarets, and the camel rides around Giza Pyramids and Jaisalmer; driving along the stunning coastline in Algarve and eating Peri, Peri chicken in Lisbon.

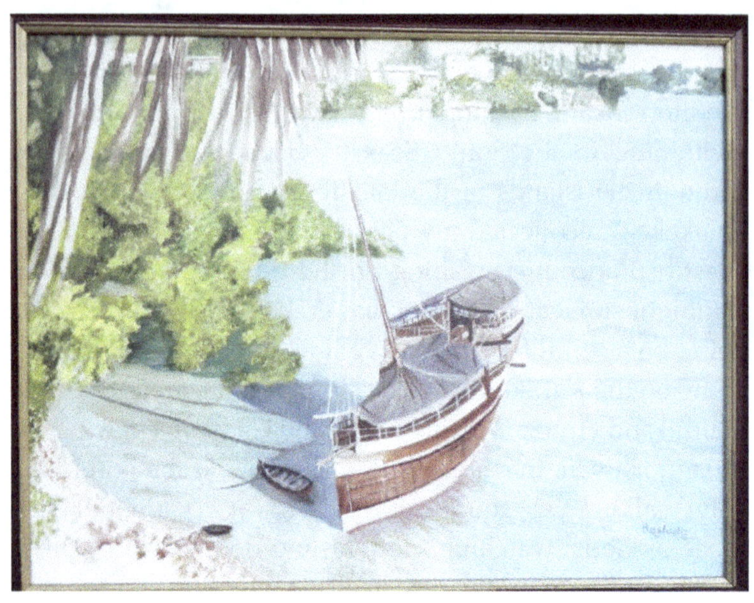

Having cancer is a demanding 24/7 business; there is the daily attention to appointments which are just for survival. During the span of chemotherapy treatments my life revolved around medical appointments e.g. blood requisition on Mondays, appointment with the oncologist to check body weight and blood work on Tuesday, Wednesday was for various classes on lymphedema, and how to cope with cancer, nutrition, chemotherapy, Look Good, Feel Better and chemo on Thursday. One hour prior to chemo, prescription medications had to be taken to prevent vomiting and nausea. There are 17 cancer care centres in Alberta and the closest one to my home required a two hour round trip drive to Tom Baker Cancer Centre. This level of activity is onerous for a cancer patient on aggressive treatment. I slept for 17-18 hours allowing my cells time to regenerate. In addition to daily medical treatment, my home-aid worker spent an hour and half ensuring I took my shower, massaged my dry skin with oils to prevent sores, helped me with exercise and did my meal prep. I declined evening service to tuck me in bed as I was usually asleep.

I shared news of my cancer with friends and relatives and received varying reactions from personal visits, to being with me during treatment, love, prayers, flowers, books, fruit baskets, healthy meal plates, special cushions for my back problems, air purifiers, diffuser and cards. My neighbours surprised me with huge planters on my patio that they regularly watered and maintained lending colour and beauty to my home. Whilst there were others who refrained from any contact. I have learnt that social connections change as some old ones crumble and new connections emerge even stronger. I have cherished and will always remember the kindness shown by varied well-wishers and sincerely pray for them. Some people come into your life as blessings, whilst others come to teach you lessons. I believe that ultimately, you must know the difference and allow your attitude to be one of solace, be a warrior, and not the victim and find inner strength for emotional, physical, and psychological well-being.

Unfortunately, telephone calls from concerned friends and relatives were too numerous, clogging voicemail and adding stress to my already fragile existence. Being on my own this stress was onerous as my love for telephone communication was never good, even when I was well. Many cancer patients totally reject any social interaction due to their low immunity and distance themselves from social media, phone or email. I would recommend that before commencing treatment, any cancer patient should inform their network of friends and relatives to refrain from calling. Depending on the treatment, one will likely be too weak to converse or respond to enquiries, as they may not realize the toll it can take to engage in conversation, let alone the same conversation with several people in a day. Instead, encourage concern to be expressed through emails, cards, flowers, fruits etc. Your voicemail has to be available for the numerous medical appointments, and messages from medical callers trying to schedule daily appointments or remind you of one. I did not have the strength, time or inclination to delete social messages and my voice mail capacity for 10 was always full. The Medical community informed me of its inability to leave messages and commenced mailing me appointment reminders. My nurse and care worker recognized my inability to exercise tougher control on social calls and deleted them to create space for medical calls.

Brain fog proved to be a menace and nuisance. Forgetting names, use of incorrect words, lapses for sentences and thoughts, offering my credit card instead of a cancer card because it was better looking was demonstrative of a total lack of understanding. In retrospect, brain fog was the cause of many funny situations on account of the wrong use of words or sentences. I was unable to say 'thank you' and instead kept saying 'love you'. The consequence was favourable as health care providers got accustomed to my endearing acknowledgement, and loudly responded 'love you too' and remembered me. Reading a magazine as I waited for my appointments was a norm. I continued this even when I was unable to read due to blurry vision, and inability to process information due to brain fog. I still held magazines pretending to read when one of the patients kindly informed me that I was holding the magazine incorrectly! A patient humorously told us how she had driven through a bank's drive through to request her prescription.

I have always prided myself for lack of anger and being in control of my emotions. Chemotherapy treatment proved to be a spoiler as my brain fog contributed to sudden uncontrollable outbursts of anger because I felt pushed or threatened. This period of sudden anger lasted for five to six weeks, and although I remember individuals who I used to lose my temper with, I have failed to apologize for my behaviour.

One of my visits to the downtown central library met with an inconvenient loss of memory on where I had parked my car. I was certain it was parked near the Ramada Plaza downtown (familiarity due to an ownership stake in the 90's). After three hours of searching and calling car park offices that closed for the weekend, the front desk at Ramada helped me realize I was in the wrong quadrant of the city based on my parking receipt. A taxi ride to the library and circling the other side of Macleod yielded no success, compelling me to call upon a friend and her cousin at a dinner party to come to my rescue. They were quick to find my car and I have never felt more foolish but equally happy to see my car!

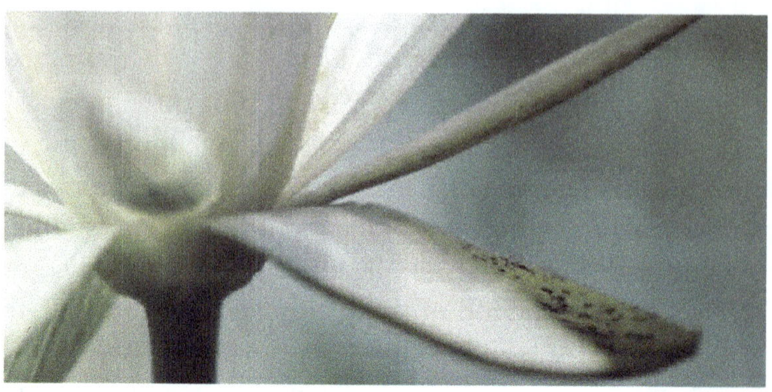

The power of positive vibes, prayers from relatives, friends, neighbours and strangers, and my faith in their prayers aided my determined fight. In waiting for a daily night show at the Grand Princess Resort in Playa Del Carmen, I identified a young 18 year old in the audience who was getting the same toxic treatment as myself at Tom Baker Cancer Centre. I eagerly raced to greet her and saw a Game boy in her hand and a perplexed frozen look suggesting she was in a severe brain fog. I exchanged a brief conversation with her mum and aunt and was grateful to God for my recovery, prayed for her well-being, and attributed my strength to the multitude of prayers.

Port Insertion

Lymph node extraction from my left hand permitted medical staff the use of my right hand for blood tests and chemotherapy infusion. After four months of enduring multiple pokes to my discoloured right hand, I became apprehensive as nurses declared veins in my right hand to be problematic. This made me a candidate for port insertion. The Medical Imaging department at South Campus Hospital provided an explanation of a port implant to be placed under my skin about 2 to 3 centimetres below my right collar bone. Discomfort from this implant was constant but proved efficient during treatment as the nurse inserted a sterile needle in the middle part of the port and removed the needle from the access site upon completion of the intravenous treatment. For weekly blood tests, blood was drawn from veins in my hand. Lesson learnt is to request a port insertion early in the process, if you have tricky veins.

Insertion and extraction of port requisitioned a blood test a few days prior and I was required to fast from midnight for both procedures. The surgeon explained the 45-minute procedure to be administered under local anesthetic and prior to inserting and extracting the port required an executed consent form. I was given a hospital gown and lay on a procedure table with local anesthetic being administered prior to inserting the port, which was amazingly smooth free of pain or discomfort. In the recovery room, I was given orange juice, coffee and a warm muffin.

Port removal required a blood test, fasting and a one-hour recovery time prior to leaving the hospital. Unfortunately, the extraction was very painful and required two nurses to hold my hands as I kept screaming despite the local numbing. In the recovery room, I was provided with coffee and a turkey sandwich but the pain of my procedure lingered. This procedure has been the worst in pain and itch to this day, eight months after the procedure. Continued symptoms of a burning itch, discomfort, and sometimes pain at the site of the stitches persists. These symptoms are not a norm and my oncologist and physician have checked the incision and unanimously indicated the stitches to be free of infection. I have since been told this is a keloid, raised scar tissue, and referred to a plastic surgeon for steroid injections to ease the pain and itching. I have been injected twice and the itching persists with a raw and angry scar. I would recommend avoiding a port if veins can accommodate the chemotherapy transfusion. In addition the needle probe at the point of insertion into the port for every infusion was painful (I used ice packs for ten minutes to numb the area prior to the needle probe). For me, port extraction has been the worst procedure through my long journey of several procedures. Other cancer patients report positive outcomes with port experience and recommend its insertion for ease in chemotherapy transfusion and report a faint to almost invisible trace of the scar from stitches.

Radiation

Understandably, refusal for radiation treatment was not a sound decision for my oncologist, Dr. Barbera, who knew better. Hence, I was invited for a second visit and met with another oncologist, Dr. Abdullah, who categorically rejected my decision and declared it as flawed. He reminded me of my long journey with diagnosis, surgery and chemotherapy and declared these efforts as incomplete without radiation. He stated with certainty that radiation treatment improved my chances of fighting cancer by 12% and not taking this final step was opening me to exposure. He was persuaded that the benefit risk ratio for taking the treatment pointed to more benefits and was convinced that my fears regarding my sister and her treatment outcomes were dated. Although he was not willing to provide any guarantees on lymphedema, he implored me to reconsider my options. Despite my displaying symptoms of lymphedema and wearing a compression sleeve to manage and cope with lymphedema symptoms, I consented to radiation. It is useful for the reader to understand that chemotherapy and radiation work in tandem with surgery and are complementary. When you embark on your journey to fight cancer you should plan and expect the three procedures.

I had been severely influenced by witnessing my sister's struggle with lymphedema from her post-surgery and radiation, and had fearfully rejected radiation initially. My journey with cancer has been similar to that of my sister in prognosis, surgery and metastasis, and am mortified at the prospect of a similar plight with lymphedema. Lymphedema is a huge swelling, heaviness, tingling, pain, discomfort and increased risk of infection.

Research indicates that between 5-30% breast cancer patients are likely to be afflicted with lymphedema on account of cancer surgery or radiation. I am part of this statistic, at risk for lymphedema in the breasts, arms, and hands due to lymph fluid accumulation. Palliative care for my sister was daunting due to lymphedema and a swollen hand 4 to 5 times her normal hand size, making any physical movement impossible. She lay on her back at all times with her hand by her side, and the nurses massaged her back for blisters. Morphine reduced her cancer pain but the swollen hand restricted any movement. I have an onset of lymphedema and have used compression garments for my hands, arms and legs despite this process being time consuming and uncomfortable. Regretfully, my arms keep growing and the compression garments no longer fit.

I commenced daily radiation treatment in the basement of Tom Baker Cancer Centre during November 2019. My treatments were delivered by Radiation Therapists who took a 3D image of the area to be treated and developed a customized treatment plan. Radiation therapy is localised using high-energy rays to kill cancer cells and destroy mutated cells remaining in the breast or armpit area after surgery. Each treatment required me to lie on my back, have my arms above my head, and the radiation was aimed at the same spot every time. This entire treatment required taking deep breaths and holding my breath to push my heart away from the chest wall and out of the treatment area.

The radiation therapists were not to be in the room and administered radiation and monitored my breathing through computers, close circuit cameras and communicated through an intercom system. Radiation for breast cancer can burn your skin to look brown. Your breast tissue may also feel firm or swollen. Radiation burns cause discomfort and require skin care during and after treatment. To ease discomfort from radiation, I wore loose cotton shirts, applied saline water and tripled the application of the recommended Glaxal moisturising cream. This spared my skin from drying, blistering or peeling.

Radiation waits were long, sometimes 30-45 minutes, and a cancer patient waiting for her treatment regularly enquired as to my satisfaction with the tattooing? She wondered as to the patterns and colour I had chosen. I was slow to understand her humour and surprised her with a beautiful bright colour floral design from a magazine and mildly complained that the process was slow and duplicating bright colours did not meet the required standard. We both laughed and found this to be a regular topic of conversation.

The mirrors in our changing room had unique and inspiring messages scrawled by an anonymous patient. I looked forward to reading these changing inspirational messages as they were reminders on focusing on results, not methods. The messages inspired positivity and synergy for patience, courage, hope and dominion over self. I loved reminders of beauty being the inner self with the human spirit providing insights and the will to act.

Completion of chemo or radiation treatments met with the tradition of a patient ringing a bell near the elevator as a celebration of completing an important benchmark in an individual's fight. It also provided for camaraderie and a distraction for the ones still receiving the treatment with the message that this phase is temporary and will pass. Upon completion of my chemotherapy treatment I did not indulge in this tradition but completion of my radiation met with a response to the contrary. More than six patients waiting for their radiation coupled with reception staff and visitors in the area gathered near the elevator and sang "Don't worry, be happy," thumping their feet and clapping their hands to:

Here's a little song I wrote
You might want to sing it note for note
Don't worry, be happy
In every life we have some trouble
But when you worry you make it double
Don't worry, be happy now

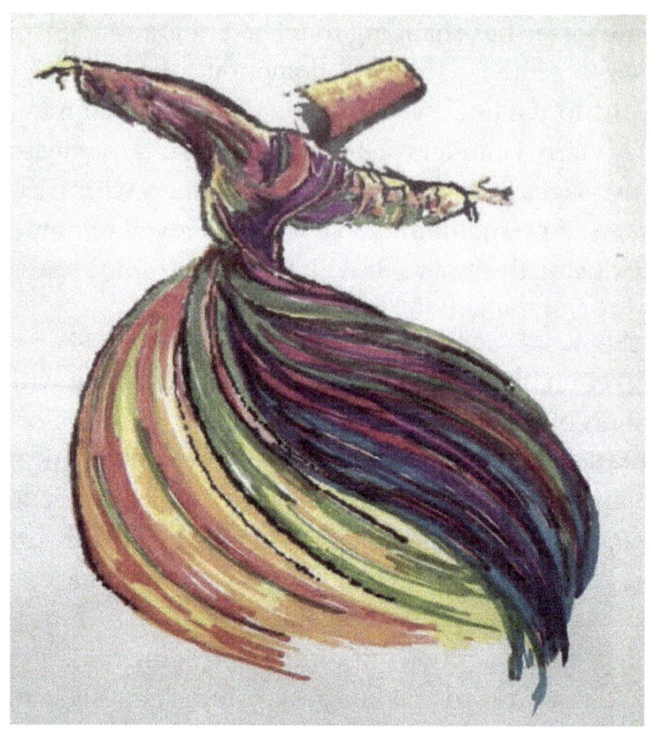

Finishing treatment was a major milestone and a good excuse to celebrate. Physically, my body was weak but emotionally I was a whirling dervish ecstatically performing pirouettes. Fourteen months of isolation due to a compromised immune system with regular prayers in the sanctity of my home met with the freedom to visit the Jamatkhana (a place for worship) to express my gratitude! My friends, Roshan and Zahir, hosted a celebratory lunch for the completion of my treatments. The company was cordial, my meal delicious, and I happily enjoyed my meal and company. I am the same person with a different lens ~ habitually, my celebrations consisted of a dinner at a restaurant, with a visit to the theatre or an entertainment hot spot. I was just as jubilant in keeping my digestive track happy in feeding it seven hours prior to retiring to bed.

Lesson being that it is important to adapt and accept changing circumstances as happiness is relative and governed by your state of mind.

The end of treatment was exciting as it marked an end to a long and somber journey of stressful daily hospital visits. This phase is difficult and complicated irrespective of whether you are surrounded by loved ones or no one. Whilst the number of people in your lives can help with resources, assurances and emotional support ~ the resilience and hopefulness can only be mustered by the person living the experience. Since age 18 my life has been independent and I prefer to be alone. There is merit in having help and support from other people, whether family, friends, religious groups, support groups, professional counselors, or others but I am firmly grounded in a belief that the journey of a soul is singular. I have upheld a modified version of independence in the face of this invidious cancer having fragmented my life – I replaced the previous unstoppable social platforms to a new norm of coping with day to day existence with remembrance of God and the noisy social norms have lost their sparkle never to return. Despite a host of services and programs, I maintained my independence in driving myself to the hospital for treatments so as not to inconvenience a well-wisher or volunteer. I am cognizant of the emotional struggles my brothers, relatives, and friends may be feeling but at this stage of life I can only look after my interests without being considered selfish.

Compassion

Receiving unconditional concern and love during my journey with cancer, I stared into an abyss of suffering and misfortune and wondered, what is compassion? And how great is this compassion? I discovered the enormity of genuine concern at every turn and in all spaces, leading me to conclude that the heart is huge and makes a difference wherever it can. I realized that I had paid lip service to the ideology of compassion as unconditional giving knows no boundaries. I had always treated people with respect and been giving, but on my terms. Having been brought up in Kenya, educated in England and having immigrated to Canada by age 22, I felt 'different'. As a new and young immigrant, I worked long hours and embraced a life of hard work, honesty, frugality, helping others in need of help, assisting families settle in their new homes but based on my convenience.

A strong work ethic for effective job performance took time, energy and showered significant success in my corporate life creating a habit for working long hours. I consoled myself for the contributions I made in enabling tourism development in the Bahamas, Cuba, Caribbean, Mexico and Florida. My executive role enabled decisions for sustainable programs for diverse cultures, skill transfers for an improved labor pool, equipment and resources for the benefit of the marginalized and assessing environmental impacts from tourism. Unfortunately, these initiatives were policy-driven and strategic, allowing little to no time for face to-face interaction in understanding the needs of the marginalized. This phase could have been balanced with more social giving for the needy, vulnerable, aged and sick.

My life was not devoid of giving, as opportunities arose from my appointments to boards and committees. As a member for religious education in the mid-70's I had the honour of initiating Saturday morning classes with its infrastructure of teachers, curriculum, programs and support teams. In the late 70's as a member of Ismaili National Council for Canada, I was provided with opportunities to be a pioneering member for Focus Humanitarian Assistance, an NGO that provided food, shelter and education for twelve hundred orphans and marginalized children in India. As a fundraiser for the opening of the Ismaili Centre, Burnaby, I became an integral part of a powerful symbol of Ismaili permanence in Canada. Subsequently, fundraising opportunities for the Aga Khan University Hospital, in Karachi, the Aga Khan Rural Support Programme in Gujarat, Gilgit and Chitral, provided for improving quality of lives for people in developing countries. In the late 90's programs for empowering Immigrant Women from Afghanistan, gave me the satisfaction of helping causes bigger than myself. It was these initial causes that falsified my thinking of having served humanity and gave me the misperception of being a humanist. It was my fight with cancer and witnessing an overwhelming power of unconditional love and compassion that I realized the true meaning of face-to-face giving. My adulthood witnessed a healthy life, extensive travel, continued education, and a good standard of living but I had short changed myself in helping the less fortunate. It took cancer to teach me the different levels of genuine caring, and a realization of true empathy, and unconditional giving. There is no time for regret but to use my fragile strength to help others even if it's not convenient.

I have no doubt that the compassionate and kind are happier and at greater peace for their virtuous qualities. Thus, I have opted to write this book to help others benefit from my journey. Excuses for inability to research due to library closures have been overcome and I have attempted an authentic version of my personal experience. I would like to share a profound excerpt from the Einstein Papers stating:

"A human being is part of a whole, called by us the "Universe," a part limited in time and space. He experiences himself, his thoughts and feelings, as something separate from the rest- a kind of optical delusion of consciousness. This delusion is a kind of prison for us, restricting us to our personal desires and to affection for a few persons nearest to us. Our task must be to free ourselves from this prison by widening our circle of compassion to embrace all living creatures and the whole of nature in its beauty."

This quote resonates with health care volunteers and workers who are focused stakeholders partnering for improved outcomes. Partnerships stretch from leading surgeons, oncologists, researchers and health care workers who lead by example in sharing knowledge and mentoring. What is it that allows these highly successful individuals to continue to care for the less fortunate and help when they live in pressurised time bubbles?

The Alberta Health Services (AHS) has introduced many initiatives to serve cancer patients effectively e.g. AHS President's Excellence award for high standards in quality improvement, innovation, collaboration and patient-centered care in 2019 was received by Provincial Breast Health. The success of these programs has been due to the patients, administrators, clinicians and front-line staff. Breast cancer patients have a plethora of resources available to help them through challenging times but the key is to know what's available and how to access these services to make a positive difference. You can benefit from drawing on a powerful blend of available resources to a practical use of them to help you enjoy greater independence. Please take solace in my example of effective use of available resources to help me in my journey. I am a single woman, living alone, new to the province, new neighbours, new physicians, and I have overcome my journey using some of these resources as my support system.

Some of the major initiatives are automatically in place with surgeons, oncologists, radiologists, nurses, primary care physicians and support staff reviewing every aspect of a breast cancer patient's journey. Waiting to meet with a health care provider for diagnosis and treatment can be harrowing and stressful but my experience provided for a seamless journey from expedited appointments, simultaneous notification to all concerned, surgery, homecare, systemic and radiation treatments, access to informative reading materials, websites and classes for additional information. The health care system's use of a best practices model provided for excellent response times and comprehensive care through the entire system of services needed. I marvel, applaud and deeply appreciate the handholding provided from the initial shock to later vulnerabilities from weakness to brain fog as debilitating conditions made better by the care provided by the health care system. My current state of independence and quality of life is owed to faith, and hope but also to the caring, kindness, prayers and good wishes by volunteers providing essential services to cancer patients. These expressions of kindness and compassion demonstrate rich wisdom and understanding the essence of life. I sincerely pray for all who have unconditionally touched my life.

I have been emotionally touched and am grateful and appreciative for the programs and resources which have motivated my independence, fending for myself and given me the resilience for my fight against cancer. For the benefit of the reader, a list of these programs and services is attached so you may avail of them based on your needs.

Programs and Services

Counselling for cancer patients to help them meet their basic needs.

Tel: 403-355-3207

- medical insurance
- income support and financial assistance
- transportation and accommodation
- disability benefits

Research and reading library for your cancer - Knowledge Resource Service Tel: 403-521-3765

Wheels of Hope - upwards of 126 volunteer drivers in Calgary help patients for treatment appointments. Tel: 1-800-263-6750 http://www.cancer.ca

Find a Wig – Canadian Cancer Society

https://canadiancancersociety.formstack.com/forms/cis_mo re_info_en

Tel: 1-888-939-3333

Written Resources by Alberta Health Services.

Guide to Tom Baker Cancer Centre, Holy Cross Centre, Peter Lougheed Centre

Breast Cancer and You A guide for women living with breast cancer. Fifth Edition

What to expect When Having Breast Surgery at the Rockyview General Hospital Nov 2018.

After Breast Cancer Surgery Range of Motion & Physical Exercise Flow Chart April, 2018

Journey through Breast Cancer Surgery

Systemic Treatment

Radiation Treatment

After Treatment

Conversations Matter

Goals of Care Designation ~ your Green Sleeve through a healthcare provider.

Cancer Related Group Classes, call 1-800-914-5665

New Patient Class Register online bit.ly/book-cancerpatiented call 1-855-258-9963 For Calgary patients please call (403) 355-3207 each session consists of 12 weekly meetings for 3 sessions per year

- For women within their first year after diagnosis of breast cancer
- For women with Stage 1-3 breast cancer

Group for Women with Metastatic Breast Cancer

Please call (403) 355-3207 On-going weekly meetings at the Psychosocial Department at Tom Baker Cancer Centre

Emotional Support

Please call (403) 355-3207. For counselling and support for you and your family and friends is available at the Department of Psychosocial Resources at the Holy Cross Site. Professional counsellors help you and your family cope with emotional, psychosocial and social stresses which often surface as a result of cancer and its treatment.

Chemotherapy Help to Manage your Treatments, Tel: (403) 521-3722

The Power of Nutrition Eating Well During Cancer Treatment – Nutrition Myths & Healthy Eating

Thinking and Memory Problems

Understanding Lymphedema How to Reduce Your Risk and Get Help. Tel: (403) 698-8169

Look Good Feel Better – Signature Steps Guide Online www.lgfb.ca Call 1-800-914-5665

Exercising for Your Life How Physical Activity May Help You. Registration not required

Living Your Best during Radiation Therapy
 Tel: (403) 521-3771

Living Your Best with Advanced, Metastatic, Chronic or Non-Curable Cancer. bit.ly/book-cancerpatiented call 1-855-258-9963 Calgary patients please call (403) 355-3207

Wellspring Cancer ~ a lifeline to cancer support offering more than 45 informed programs.

<u>www.wellspringcalgary.ca</u> Wellspring Calgary a charitable organization with locations at Carma House and Randy O'Dell House offering more than 45 programmes:

- Groups Educational Programmes
- Expressive Arts
- Movement and Meditation
- Caregiving and Self-care
- Money Matters
- Speakers Series
- Kid Friendly
- Young Adult Connection
- Energy Sessions
- Peer Support
- External Support Cancer Groups

<u>www.wellspringcalgary.ca</u>

Tel: (403) 521-5292

Living with Cancer

Surgery, chemotherapy and radiation have helped in restricting cancer growth but I have not beaten cancer. Warnings of being a prime candidate for a recurring cancer bring chilling thoughts of dire treatment months. Oncologists do set goals for cancer patients to stay alive long enough to take advantage of the advances in science. Getting the diagnosis of cancer can be life altering and to beat the disease through treatment is triumphant but to have it recur can be devastating. I am cautiously hopeful and optimistic for a quality of life free of sickness, treatments, hospital visits and suffering. I would like to obliterate the cancer chapter and get back to resuming life to spreading awareness, volunteering in an advisory capacity for cancer patients.

It is my understanding that current screening practices can detect recurring cancer only after it reaches high levels of metastasis. CT scans lack the resolution to detect remnant cells while blood tests have a resolution limit to detect cancer when millions of cells are present. Let's hope that science innovation can proactively introduce procedures and equipment, capable of detecting recurrence before it reaches high levels of metastasis.

When medical professionals suggest that you live life, make the most of every day and be happy, it is based on their knowledge of a probable relapse. Arguably, I am convinced that when you have cancer, the journey is about you, the need to look after yourself, and embrace the new you. Being comfortable with your natural self allows control designating you as the driver and not the passenger. It has been the toughest journey of my life and the best lesson provider for adaptability to the new reality of changed circumstances. In addition to your medicine in a bottle, take care of yourself, find joy in pain, be independent, separate fact from fiction, meditate, assess what is important and remain at peace in a calming space, be positive, and sometimes have the strength to help others on a similar journey. For me, it is not the fear of death that is troubling but the uncertainty of the events that precede it. If only we could move into the future in a time machine to understand what it offers?

Treatment of cancer affects both the body and mind and the physical changes accompanying the treatment. You will be fatigued and unable to cope with basic chores, your physical appearance will change as your self-image and many things prior to your treatments will increasingly matter less. Experiencing weight gain linked to chemotherapy, different steroids or hormone therapies can be a struggle but live in the moment and do not allow physical appearances to concern you. Most visible are changes related to hair loss and weight gain. Hair loss is a temporary issue, and can regrow once you finish your treatment. My thoughts have been bulleted for your benefit:

- Much as I hate being afflicted by cancer, it's the mortality that has provided a fresh perspective on relationships and an understanding for what matters. My weaknesses and frail physical strength have slowed my pace and taught me to prioritize things that are important and need to be accomplished whilst my vulnerabilities have removed pretensions and unfolded a closer truth to who I am.

- I have been a warrior in following the health team recommendations. I cannot explain nor understand how I survived my gruelling 14 months with the malignant demon through every phase of my journey. I am convinced it has been due to prayers, faith, hope, courage, strength, calmness and intrinsic human survival instinct. My family, relatives and friends with their prayers and hope gave me the strength to fight with reassurances that pain and suffering is limited to the physical body but not the spirit. With certainty my spirit has not only gained strength but I have become a better human being with patience, endurance, maturity and caring for humanity. It's not the physical body but the spirit's connection to the mind that has made me a warrior to muster strength for the fight.

- A visit to my hairdresser preceded the treatment phase with a request for a stubble haircut as opposed to getting shaved to avoid ingrown hair and an itchy scalp. Upon receipt of the strongest cancer treatment drug, my bald head was vogue in the chemo wards. Canadian Cancer Society donated a real hair wig which I never wore…..this wig was not me and I felt phony, uncomfortable and my scalp was irritated … My bald head was easy maintenance and not having to shampoo and dry my hair was a perfect solution at a time of low energy. I bought myself three caps but was gifted a dozen in a variety of shapes and colours to match my attire and winter coats. By the end of January my hair commenced its visible growth and in February soft salt and pepper curls allowed me a different but appealing look. It's becoming, and age appropriate!

- My body shape or size is of no consequence and the thought of reconstructive surgery or use of prostheses sounds unnecessary. My chest to the left side is numb to senses and I have stitches as a symbol of my fight but being alive and pain free is more important. Cancer has attacked my body but not my spirit. I still want to laugh, exchange jokes, dance virtually and appreciate nature. I have been cured of being self-conscious based on how others see me but am content to be who I am.

- If physical appearance is important then I would suggest arranging for the following in advance, for the services you deem appropriate:

- hair stylist

- makeup artist

- Reiki master

- massage therapist

- Latin dance instructor

- personal trainer

- I am a strong adherent to the principle of peace with zero tolerance for violence, even if it's news or a documentary. Chemotherapy treatments have altered my choice for movies and entertainment to romantic comedies as I personalize scenes of violence and become the target to getting shot, abused or insulted.

- I used to sleep 16-18 hours and had a bitter palate. I was fatigued with no energy for physical activity, and my weight remained constant irrespective of my eating habits and sedentary lifestyle. Upon completion of my chemotherapy, I slept 10-12 hours and six months after my treatment my sleeping patterns are becoming erratic. I generally sleep 8-10 hours and sometimes 6-8 hours.

- My digestive tract is sluggish, compelling me to eat food by 4 PM to enable digestion. I have been a food lover but now I reject certain foods and display preference for different foods e.g. I was accustomed to coconut water. Now I reject coconut water and substitute it with ginger ale. My love for proteins is dwindling as my craving for carbohydrates (french fries, bread, rice, potatoes, pasta, chips etc.) meets with non-stop consumption. I need a plan toward better eating and a disciplined work-out regimen.

- I am adept at coping and managing with isolation as my 14 month journey with surgery and treatments confined me to a solitary and sedentary life due to a compromised immune system. Now Covid-19 has imposed a further 6-8 months or more of self-isolation and social distancing which I accept without any complaints. My self-isolation has allowed for this book to be written, more time for reflection, initiating projects to occupy my time and attention to help others.

- Cancer has taught me to live each day as if it's my last. Two years ago I would have scoffed at any suggestion that I would write this book but now I need to share my message with others in the hope that they may benefit from reading it. Writing a book is a complicated process of writing, editing, and publishing which is time consuming, costly and daunting. My willingness to undergo these challenges comes from giving support and strength to others who may benefit from my experience.

- Waiting for my treatment, I often talked with other cancer patients who were miserable and complained about the side-effects of the treatment or not receiving the expected empathy from their family members. I reflected that a complaining mind does not appear at peace, and I, with a grateful heart, am at peace. Of what avail are misery and complaints in walking a journey you have to walk, leading me to conclude that my attitude of being calm and grateful for what I have must be contributing to my peace.

- Before my cancer diagnosis I was given to thinking about opportunities and was immersed in a busy life with no time to cherish all that nature offers. The median life expectancy for my sort of metastatic breast cancer is five years and with this immortality natural wonders are hypnotic, mesmerising and a great source for reflection. Thanking God has been a routine process but now there is a difference in my attitude and emotions. I thank God for giving me the opportunity to reflect on my environment and admire the sun rays, moon, stars, sunsets, sunrises, mountains and natural wonders.

- A list of fiduciary responsibilities has been itemized, prioritized and I am grateful for this opportunity. I have paid my leases upfront, saleable assets have been sold to activate my revised bucket list wishes.

- Equipped with the knowledge that I cannot wave a wand and miraculously be cancer free, I acknowledge my struggles. I am determined to be a good stakeholder and cooperate with the medical team and use my pain free 'cope and manage' situation to attempt a bucket list of things to do.

In writing this book I share my reality with others walking a similar journey to inspire an attitude of hope, fight, cope, manage and lead as normal a life. Being diagnosed with cancer is not a death sentence as early detection provides for survival rates and many exceed 5 years+ to be proclaimed cancer free. This book is to provide understanding and empower those dealing with metastatic breast cancer to find strength in the esoteric part of their being. There's no cure for metastatic breast cancer yet, but it's treatable. Some women live for many years after a diagnosis of Stage 4 breast cancer. I am petrified but stoic about my breast cancer's high likelihood of traveling to the brain, lungs or bones, but I enjoy the moment and want to be free of this unpredictability. The saga of complicated events unrolling is ongoing and will continue.

My family has been at war against an aggressive cancer and my mother and sister fought a valiant battle but ultimately lost to the disease. Are we any further ahead to 50 years ago when I lost my mother, and 25 years ago when I lost my sister to breast cancer? My mother died within three months and my sister within 24 months. Having spent 14 months undergoing surgery and treatments to a localised area I too dance with the looming prospect of recurrence and meeting the malignant demon with amplified lethality head-on. I ponder if my mum and sister were better off than me in having a shorter fight? This thought is not to undermine the kindness given by my surgeon, oncologist, radiologists, nurses and all stakeholders in the hope that treatment given will make me cancer free. They come equipped with kindness, compassion, programs, services, new treatments and therapies, **but they cannot make it go away**. The skeptic in me rationalizes that many of the drugs and treatment options currently under development won't be available for years' and even though researchers allege a cure for breast cancer to be imminent unless these cures meet with immediate release many lives could be lost.

The fight I speak of is not only to fight the disease but to fight for a cure. It's a pity that despite the best concentration of medical and scientific expertise and limitless resources the struggle for a cure has met with failure. Given these circumstances, it is not surprising for cancer patients and their families to angrily assert that pharmaceutical companies caring for profits from expensive chemotherapy treatments and other related drugs is an obstacle to research for a cure.

This conspiracy theory does not win my support. What is the counter argument to this claim? The pharmaceutical empire globally comprises 10-20 thousand companies competitively seeking a cure, with scientists working to become famous in finding a cure for any of the cancers, which is likely to amass billions of dollars. I am troubled about unsatisfactory outcomes in meeting cures for cancer. It's a pity that the journey with cancer is a tale of suffering, pain and death for many; it's a pity that research has had an inordinate amount of time with no solutions; it's a pity that exorbitant financial resources for research have brought no concrete solutions apart from an awareness of the inherent complexities.

Recent exposure to the Covid-19 pandemic and the global community uniting to find a vaccine against the horrid pandemic is a fine example of combined global efforts to fight the monstrous disease. It is time for initiatives and actions to be implemented globally in finding a cure for cancer. Too many decades of failure to find successful solutions have been tolerated and we must appoint a leader who will demand firm action, responsibility, accountability, and advocacy on a global basis with critical paths for action. There are no boundaries for this disease and the best leader who can champion a cause to fight cancer has to be identified with the best qualifications for a strategic approach for successful outcomes. A cure is vital in light of the looming prediction that 40% of the Canadian population is likely to have cancer in the next 15 years.

By no means should my reflections suggest regret at the life I have lived. In fact, I am grateful for all I have achieved and having lived life on my terms and as best as I could. But it is human to reflect, and I think it a pity that it was cancer that awakened my soul to lose pretence; cancer exposed the new me. It is normal to indulge in reflections of your life and would you do things differently if given an opportunity? I would respond to my times and circumstances no differently than I did at academic accreditations, material accomplishments, acculturation, integration, assimilation, mannerisms, language dexterity, clothes, life-style, friends and more that added value as each single event was experiential and taught me lessons.

My journey with this dreaded malignant demon, who the oncologists described as tricky, and I as cunning and wicked, has allowed me to assume a deeper focus, change in mind-set and minimized conditionality. It's a relief that I have always been spiritual and a humanist giving generously, but may be not generously enough. It's a pity that deep contemplation and honest assessment has come due to cancer. I am grateful for this wake-up call for my virtues to emerge in planning finances for humanistic giving and basic needs for an unpredictable life. Is it the face of mortality brought about by cancer that has ushered this change? My spirit wants to attain a life-time of living and giving in whatever time I may have and genuinely believe that my decisions will be richer because of life experiences. I had planned to do so much and had deferred many action items for retirement years. Lesson learnt...not to procrastinate and live life fully for every moment. I realize the strength of this lesson with my compromised physical strength that no longer permits a life of serving and giving as the future becomes a pragmatic response to coping with reality.

Determining the effectiveness of my surgery and treatment lies in the screening and follow-up appointments. However, Covid-19 has intrusively disrupted appointments until further notice. The anxiety and fear of recurrence with the probability that the cancer might never go away completely is like a recurring nightmare forcing me to accept unpredictability. I sit in my conflict zone patiently waiting for my follow-up appointments as I continue to live life with a new normalcy.

'God grant me the serenity to accept the things I cannot change, Courage to change the things I can, and Wisdom to know the difference'. Reinhold Niebuhr

I am human and have faced many of life's daunting challenges with cancer being the worst. I am grateful for an anchoring force called spirituality that has brought strength, endurance and stability.

Spirituality

Spirituality is not a luxury, something for people who have nothing else to do but sit around and meditate. In fact, it is the lack of spirituality in daily life that is causing the breakdown and destruction of our planet and our civilization.

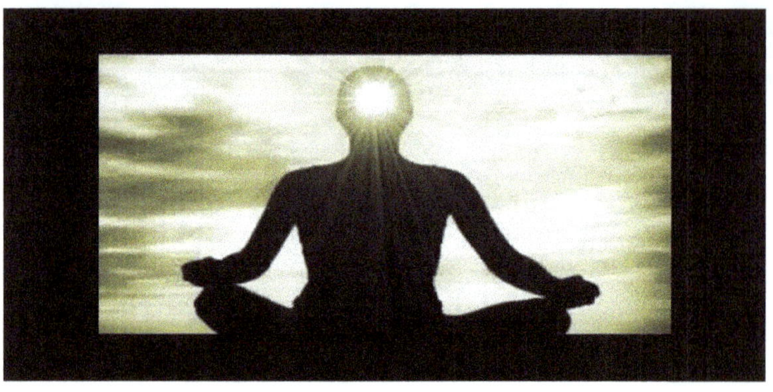

I introduce this chapter as spirituality has been an anchoring force and of enormous help in my fight against cancer, as you may have already surmised. The meaning of spirituality has developed and expanded over time with various definitions but in its simplest description, it is connecting with a bigger force than yourself to result in positive emotions such as peace, awe, contentment, and gratitude. Throughout the ages, all major faiths enable individuals to connect to the Divine as human beings have existential questions related to the meaning and purpose of life. I am convinced that in developing a strong spirit you will weather your ill-health with greater acceptance and ease. A counsellor at Foothills informed me that patients afflicted by cancer experience spirituality as different from others. Generally, patients turn to the spiritual side to help them navigate rough waters, knowing that many have taken this journey before. But even for those afflicted, spiritual feelings vary as for some it may weaken, whilst for others it may strengthen or play no role. It may challenge long-held beliefs as people living with cancer feel spiritual distress, let down by their faith and question their relationship with God. This fatal illness can usher uncertainty to your ideas, change your beliefs, play havoc with your peace of mind.

Spiritual moments can occur when one is close to nature, art, a loved one or when following a religious tradition. Spiritual beliefs are varied, diverse and nurtured in different ways. Spirituality is a dimension of your life experiences and can be strengthened based on your worldview. The key is to develop and strengthen your spirit to bring a sense of calm and serenity during your challenging times. I believe that every person has a spiritual dimension with certain beliefs and values connecting them to a deeper meaning of reality; thus it is a broad concept involving a personal search for meaning in life. In Muslim traditions, examples of spiritual search can be found in diverse Muslim musical forms, art, literature, with varied genres and interpretations.

You may draw inspiration from this quote:

"In judging our progress as individuals we tend to concentrate on external factors such as one's social position, influence and popularity, wealth and standard of education……But internal factors may be even more crucial in assessing one's development as a human being. Honesty, sincerity, simplicity, humility, pure generosity, absence of vanity, readiness to serve others – qualities which are within easy reach of each soul – are the foundation of one's spiritual life" Nelson Mandela

My spiritual disciplines stem from the perspective of a Shia Ismaili Muslim, a follower of His Highness Prince Karim Aga Khan, 49th descendant of Prophet Muhammad (pbuh), Imam of the Ismailis and provider of secular, religious and spiritual guidance to his 15 million followers who reside in over 25 countries. The Shia tradition - is rooted in the complementarity between intellect and faith. Despite a life-time search for answers, contemplation, staunch faith in God as my confidante, advisor, counsel, and best friend, I am plagued with many unanswered questions on searching for purpose and meaning and share Rumi's questions:

Every day I meditate upon this, and every night I groan

Why is my own existence to myself the least known?

Whence have I come, why this coming here?

Where to must I go, when will my home to me be shown?

I am in desperate awe, why was I ever created?

Jalaluddin Rumi

I wonder if humanity exists in a cosmic house of mirrors and what seems to be real is an illusion. Is it possible that the past, present and future make up one moment making only the present really count? If material achievement does not bring fulfillment then it must be spiritual connection which brings peace and serenity? Yes, you have your being in God and God as your Creator has breathed a spark into you, and connection to this link may be the purpose of life.

"We can't help being thirsty, moving toward the voice of water. Milk drinkers draw close to the mother. Muslims, Christians, Jews, Buddhists, Hindus, shamans, everyone hears the intelligent sound and moves with thirst to meet it."

Jalaluddin Rumi

Rumi's poems help me understand the inner depths of my consciousness, the nature of being human while yearning for the Divine, and to prioritize what is important in my life. His significance in history is not just in Sufi Islam, as he has touched millions of others, and is one of the most-read poets in the West...perhaps more so than in Muslim societies. I resonate more in my private spiritual search with secular speeches and Farmans made by the Aga Khan to the Ismaili community. The Imam has stressed the use of the intellect, to accompany our personal search, both to live our lives fully and ethically, and for faith to be understood rationally.

Despite meditation and observing my daily obligatory prayers, affliction with cancer has brought the realization that reflection to the deeper spiritual dimension of life was tepid prior to cancer. My faith tells me that struggle is the meaning of life which provides strength and patience to fight this adversity and a deeper reflection to thoughts about my parents' lives and their devotion to faith, their actions, decisions and worldviews...and how they have shaped my personality. I remain influenced by my formative upbringing despite living in different times with a communication revolution that entertains multiple voices on any subject, often opposed to my own views.

Based on my Imam's guidance, spirituality is a source of comfort, companionship, strength, tolerance, endurance, patience and intensified my quest to better understand this source of strength. It is spirituality that has been the catalyst for my change and provided strength during my times of uncertainty. I have meditated since the age of 13 and believe that it is this process of development, akin to physical, intellectual, emotional or moral, that has been my source of strength. Shams Tabriz, a philosopher and teacher of Rumi, stated that the soul unlike the intellect is in actuality imperfect but with great potentiality. Encouraged by this thought and staunch faith in guidance from the Imam, simplifies the purpose of life to knowing oneself and reflecting upon the environment.

"The Divine Intellect, 'Aql-i Kull, both transcends and informs the human intellect. It is this intellect which enables man to strive towards two aims dedicated by the Faith: that he should reflect upon the environment Allah has given and that he should know himself. It is the light of intellect which distinguishes the complete human being from the human animal and developing that intellect requires free enquiry."

His Highness the Aga Khan, Aga Khan University Inauguration Address, Karachi, November 11, 1985

The Covid-19 pandemic has allowed us to reflect on our relationship with the environment. As many economies have slowed the world has witnessed improved air and water quality creating a correlation between human impact and quality of our environment. Thinking of the environment is complex as one exercises less control on the existence and interaction of living and non-living things. Like spirituality, reflecting on the environment meets with diverse opinions. In simple terms the environment is everything that surrounds us and affects our ability to live on - water, air, agricultural and pastoral landscapes and all the resources we humans use.

Can we as individuals make a difference? Yes. If every individual takes their personal responsibilities seriously to bring a collective change in outcome. The Aga Khan has repeatedly reminded us of our role as stewards of Divine creation and in his speech to the Royal Architectural Institute of Canada in 2013, he said:

"For our faith constantly reminds us to observe and be thankful for the beauty of the world and universe around us, and our responsibility and obligation, as good stewards of God's creation, to leave the world in a better condition than we found it......The future will present us with ever-evolving architectural challenges - urbanization, water management, air pollution, protection from manmade and natural hazards and the efficient use of limited resources"

How can we care for the environment in our daily lives?

A complete stop in using plastic and substituting it with recyclable materials would provide a healthy start to helping our environment. We could plant herbs in the kitchen and vegetable gardens in our backyards, freezing extras for consumption in the winter. Modifying our behaviours to buying local, reducing use of car and air travel to minimize our carbon footprint. We could consider eating less meat, four ounces three times a week, is recommended by nutritionists for cancer patients, and mindfully reducing our consumption of resources as everything impacts our environment.

The Aga Khan's son, Prince Hussain, in 2019 at the Resilient Housing Challenge in Geneva, spoke of natural disasters increasing in frequency and severity in mountainous and coastal areas. He spoke of glacial lake outburst floods that wipe away people's homes and livelihoods. In 2018, Prince Aly Muhammad Aga Khan in his short film, "Close to Home," created an awareness of the perseverance of communities in Northern Pakistan in the face of natural disasters. In addition, global warming due to greenhouse gas emissions and deforestation is threatening sustainable life-styles for humanity pressing the urgent need to find renewable energy sources.

Our current environmental problems of growing population, human consumption, climate change, air pollution, deforestation, rural shift of people to urban cities, and acid rain suggest the overall condition of our planet to be unhealthy. In lay-person terms, my simple knowledge surmises that solutions will have to be holistic, integrated and global in context. Action from global international entities, governments, and civil society are warranted due to recurrent crises that are global in scope. The voice of logic suggests that civil society ultimately determines quality of life for continued and sustainable change.

Reflections on the complexities of my environment overwhelm me, allowing a graceful shift to attempting an honest self-assessment. Phew...my initial thoughts of knowing myself have radically changed as a stringent scrutiny brought numerable facets that had never crossed my radar screen as I compartmentalized and measured overall emotions, empathy and generosity.

- Emotional intelligence is related to understanding, and managing my emotions to cultivate a positive state of mind to recognize something larger than myself. There are several components to undertaking this assessment and a further in-depth examination revealed several components that have been missed. This mammoth task is incomplete and I am work in progress.
- My empathy meter provided the ability to understand and share the feelings of another but from their point of view. I still need a lot of work.
- Generosity has opened my heart for the welfare of others but I am still selfish and need to practice greater giving as I have far more than the poor in this world.

A superficial and cursory assessment suggests I am malleable to greater generosity, compassion, am positive, free of gossip, envy, leading a moral and ethical life. I compare my feelings to a savings account where I comfortably draw on over five decades of faith. I cannot explain the mystery for the synergy of spiritual strength which suddenly entered my life and has allowed me to be more grateful and compassionate than before. Facing difficulties has helped me better appreciate Divine help, as I compare the difference in myself prior to cancer and now that I fight the disease. Since my affliction, spiritual growth has been pronounced with a deeper trust that Allah will ultimately do what is in my best interest and I submit, surrender and trust the Divine absolutely, irrespective of the outcome, irrespective of where this takes me, four months from now, eight months from now, or in two years.

Normal day to day concerns have taken a back seat and started to fade out of my mind-space substituting these for concerns of screening medical appointments, quiet life-style, praying, meditating, and expressing my gratitude for the abounding kindness experienced. Being a single woman, I have always valued independence, and now for the first time I am willing to compromise my independence as I depend on kind people to do things for me. It's as if I am tasting life for the first time and am fearlessly embracing the next chapter recognizing that I am powerless to control anything.

Many individuals remind me to remain positive, and I appreciate their comments with a silent evaluation of my health card and my faith. Science is based on fact and predicts a long survival rate if there is no recurrence. It cannot predict if a recurrence is possible and for me a quality of life is of greater importance than a life full of treatment, suffering and anguish.

 In my conversations with God, I reflect on the compatibility of science and faith and acknowledge a higher power to whom I am connected granting me the strength, optimism and hope that scientists will find a cure, and that research will soon provide a quality of life to help many who are afflicted. But above everything, my faith is accepting of the Divine plan, and I submit to whatever it may unfold as my life's journey. I pray for the benefit of those afflicted and to be afflicted that a cure is announced soon. The impact of having and living with cancer with its physical scars, mental recollections of pain, suffering, mortality and the emotional toll of knowing you are living with a killer can never be erased.

Embarking Once Again on a New Journey

Shamshadbegum Asaria

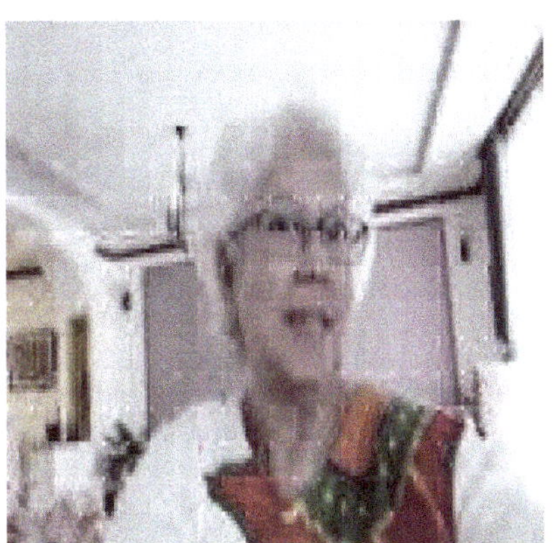

In the month of May of 2013, I was diagnosed with adenocarcinoma of the left lung, here in Nairobi, at the Aga Khan University Hospital, under the care of Dr. Nadeem Sheikh. I was explained about the disease and informed that it was diagnosed late because it was already Stage 4 Cancer.

A rug was pulled from under my feet, but also there was a sense of urgency to deal with this disease and the rush to make the right contacts, doctors, hospitals, appointments and so on. A fast journey was to begin in search of the treatment of cancer, the physical healing and therefore the feelings must be silenced for now. There was no time to lick the wound; in fact I just felt numb. My husband and I spent a quiet, sleepless night at the hospital, numb and afraid to talk. The universe started aligning with our thoughts and angels began to walk into my new reality providing support and advice at every crossroad.

Based on my nephew's recommendations, a doctor in cancer research in Michigan, and another expert opinion from an oncologist in Atlanta, I readied for my trip to Vancouver. Choice of Vancouver as our destination was predicated not only on great medical treatment available at the British Columbia Cancer Agency (BCCA), but presence of family in Vancouver and moral support we would have. From the onset, I was mindful of my husband's needs, Hassan, as a primary caregiver, to have his family and friends nearby. Scheduling appointments was very efficient and expedient allowing access to General Practitioner, Dr. Mumtaz Ali, whom I met on the second day after arriving in Vancouver and Dr. Janessa Laskin, an Oncologist a couple of days later. Dr. Laskin was accommodating and gave me hope and assurance with many options. Under her supervision and guidance, I did four cycles of chemotherapy and five radiations in all. Dr. Laskin was very clear in explaining to me that there was no cure for this cancer but with the correct treatment it could be managed for a certain time.

I returned to Nairobi in October 2013 with strict instructions to stay very closely connected to an oncologist. The doctor indicated to Hassan that I would have one year to sixteen months to live at the most. Of course, this was based on the statistics they had for a Stage 4 cancer such as mine. As luck would have it, I was connected to Dr. Asim Jamal Sheikh, in Nairobi, at the Aga Khan Hospital. He suggested a treatment called "Maintenance Chemo" with a drug called Pemetrexed (Alimta). This treatment would add two months of life after every administration and if my body adapted to it. Hence, began my second journey with cancer. I stayed on Alimta from November, 2013 to November, 2017! I was almost symptom free and at times I did not even think that I had this dreadful disease called cancer. Dr. Jamal was happy with my response to the treatment. However, the inevitable happened, the cancer cells became clever and the drug stopped working. The initial reduction in the lung tumor was erased and the tumor became active and grew in size.

I knew I was to embark on my third journey. The doctor suggested we do a CT PET scan and then figure out another set of treatments to manage the cancer. This began to look like a "Pandora Box," put your hand in and pull out a trick to confuse the clever cancer cells. I was happy to know that somewhere there were clever doctors working hard to create more tricks to beat the cancer cells. Bless their Hearts! A conference call between oncologists familiar with my condition and treatments, resulted in a trip to India as at that time a CT PET scan was not available in Nairobi. Ensuing discussions between doctors in Nairobi and India suggested Targeted Immunotherapy in the area of checkpoint inhibitors, and the drug suggested was Nivolumab (OpDivo). This short interlude started in January of 2018 to be concluded in May of 2020.

Exactly seven (7) years later, May, 2020 the new CT PET scan showed activity in the growth of tumor size and a new lesion in the spine at C7, the last cervical bone of the neck and a tricky location. This explained the shooting pain from my armpit radiating to the elbow and the stiffness and pain in the neck and upper shoulders. My oncologist suggested some radiation to C7. However, the radiation oncologist, Dr. Farrok Karsan requested more specific information from the BCCA regarding previous radiation done, if any, at C7 because with nerves coming out from there it could be tricky, if over radiated, could lead to some sort of paralysis. Dr. Karsan is a very gentle and kind oncologist exercising great caution and absolute care.

I am scheduled for an ultrasound biopsy, for samples for retests of the biomarkers such as EGFR and ALK and some new tests such as ROS and New Generation Medical Treatments, etc. These tests had to be outsourced to Dr. Khuzaima Mama in Mumbai. With the Covid-19, the courier services are offering limited services, and working with limited hospitals presenting challenges to an already tough situation. The Aga Khan Hospital Histology head, assured me that the tests will make it to their main laboratory in Mumbai through Metropolis Laboratory in Nairobi. Fortunately, Dr. Khuzaima Mama efficiently rushed the test results to my doctor. Introduction to Dr. Mama was serendipitous. While we were in Ahmedabad in India, an email from our dear friends the Nimji's suggested we get in touch with Dr. Mama, an oncologist who specializes in liver and pancreas, and renowned for treating Steve Job''s (Apple) when Steve was diagnosed with pancreatic cancer. Dr. Mama went out of his way from the goodness of his heart and for no monetary gain. In Mumbai, Dr. Mama took me to see another very busy expert oncologist at 11 p.m. at night for another opinion. A truly very humble and good human being, of whom, I am proud to call a friend. He stays connected and checks up on me regularly.

As for my fourth journey, and further treatments, I do not know right now what is to be offered to me from the Pandora's Box. I believe it may be the second line of defense chemotherapy. I just hope it does not have the same side effects as the first line of defense chemotherapy I received in Canada – nausea, vomiting, hair loss, sleepless nights, fatigue, etc. I have been given pain killers to manage pain while I wait to start my treatment.

In all this time, Hassan has stood by me and has given me his support and helped me to stay stress free, for which I am very grateful and consider myself very lucky and fortunate. Allah has sent me many blessings in the form of spouse, doctors, family and friends and has always seemed to connect me to the right people at the right time, like Zahir Popat, our most valued friend, who was there with me from the beginning of my journey in Vancouver and has continued to be with me in this entire journey so far and has been there for Hassan too, in his journey with prostate cancer, which is now in complete remission by the grace of God.

Throughout my journey, what has kept coming home is the fact that there are many kind, warm, generous, and loving people. It has been a source of hope and inspiration to me and has given me that optimism and trust that, at every crossroad in my life, I have met with knowledgeable experts directing and guiding me to doctors and cutting edge treatments. I am reminded of my very brief and chance meeting with a very brave cancer patient who gave me her hair wig during my first cycle of chemotherapy. In spite of her horrendous experience, she was so full of life, and so optimistic about my journey, she even did a dance jig in her excitement in the middle of the street where I met her. She left me with a very profound message. She told me to be that innocent child that puts her trusting hand in her mother's when crossing the street for the oncoming traffic.

This message has been engraved in my heart and I have never forgotten it. Bless her soul!

The line of angels is forever increasing and I am humbled every day. All the love and kindness reminds me of a quote by Imam Ali, "The body is purified by water, the ego is purified by tears, the intellect is purified by knowledge and the soul is purified by love". During this pandemic, Hassan and I have managed to stay safe and home and play cards on the weekends. I have spent time practicing on the harmonium, have managed to get the notes of one song completed, and can now play and sing the notes on the instrument. Music for the soul! I have used my artistic talent to create some costume jewelry to dress up for my doctor's appointments. My daily yoga exercises have helped me to be able to cross my legs again in a lotus position (almost but not quite, after breaking both the femur bones in 2015, a fall from the escalator in a shopping mall). Above all, I cherish my time in the wee hours of the morning, when I sit in peace and contemplation, remembering my maker.

I am also doing some useful things too. I have formed a team with three other like- minded friends to form a The Health and Wellness Group. We organize meetings with a group of interested people, at which I share my research on herbal remedies, we invite experts to talk on various supporting medicines, lifestyle changes, exchanging healthy tips for boosting the immunity, show solidarity and support to other patients and encouraging them to step forward and share. In my above endeavor, Chatur Group, prominent owners of some hotels and businesses in Nairobi, adopted us by offering a complimentary conference room with all the facilities for our meeting and refreshments, and snacks to boot. Need I say more? The list is endless of all the wonderful people who have touched my life and have given me the will to live and fight, to help others in order to help myself, to radiate my energy to help vibrate another overwhelmed soul who has just had his or her carpet pulled from under their feet.

I am not stressed in any way. In fact I am very content and happy and at peace with myself. I am prepared for whatever comes my way. Not once in this journey did I ask "Why me?" Also, I am very proactive and certainly going to put out a fight for as long as I can. However, I am also realistic and know that at the end of the day, the cancer cells will mutate again and become clever against every drug administered. Only Allah knows how much longer I will hold out. I hope my journey and the will to fight is an inspiration to many as I share how far I have come and am willing to fight further. We all have our own journeys, easy for some and very difficult for others. I hope that by sharing this very personal story of mine, I will have contributed to your zest for living, for putting up a fight in your area of weakness and for moving on, on your journey with ease.

My prayers are for everyone's journey to be easy, filled with joy and happiness, direction and guidance, fulfilling, enriched with spiritual bliss and to have many, many blessings, grace and peace. Ameen!

Surviving Cancer

by Roshan Hemani

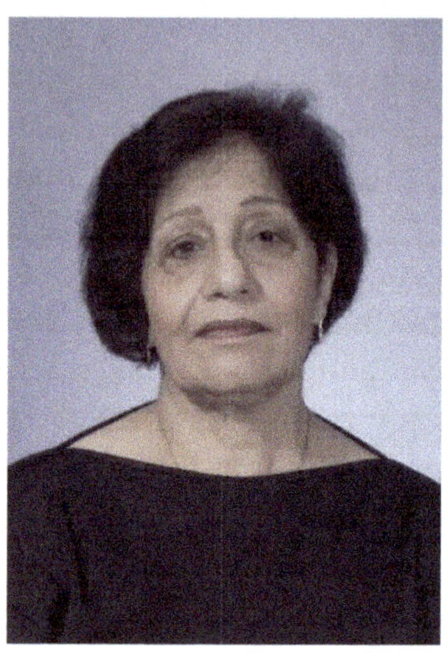

I am Roshan Hemani, cancer survivor enjoying a normal and fulfilling life as any 75 year old person can expect. This tale of fighting cancer to being a survivor started in September 2012 when I turned 67, and I submitted to a regular annual mammogram in Regina before my scheduled trip to Tanzania. I was elated to have been given a volunteer assignment to plant trees on the site of the future Aga Khan University in Arusha. My excitement at the opportunity to combine my retirement with a passion for horticulture in service to a worthwhile cause was a dream come true and a precious moment in my life. I visualized my creative contribution to the project with zest and research to ensure aesthetically pleasing outcomes.

Whilst in Arusha, I received a call from my radiographer in Regina requesting a history of my previous mammograms to analyse a new growth detected in my left breast. This matter met with quick attention as I have a maternal history of cancer. My mother, only sister, three aunts and four cousins have battled cancer. A review of previous mammograms warranted further investigation and resulted in a specialized vacuum biopsy to understand the detected growth. These circumstances prompted my return to Regina for more tests.

Unfortunately, the new growth was pronounced as cancerous with a choice of a lumpectomy or a mastectomy. Consulting with friends in the medical profession resulted in unanimous recommendations for mastectomy due to my family history. My husband was strongly supportive, purporting we needed a radical solution to our conundrum. In my state of shock I reluctantly surrendered to this decision.

In hindsight, this decision was the best as although my cancer was a Stage 1 (based on size) it was a Grade 3 (based on its maturity). Hormone testing indicated Her2 to be active and very aggressive but all other indicators were in my favour. My early detection and lymph nodes having been clear was indicative that there was no spread of cancer. Equipped with these favourable news my appointment with the oncologist was scheduled.

Her2 and the aggressive nature of my hormonal disposition, suggested that I undergo an aggressive regime of six chemotherapy treatments at three week intervals, and I was prescribed a Chemo cocktail of three drugs. In addition, I was required to continue my chemo for a period of one year with one of the three drugs specifically to control Her2 hormone. This treatment took a full year and lasted through to the end of 2013. I was warned and mentally prepared for hair loss and nausea as side effects of the treatment.

What I was ill-prepared for was sleep-deprivation. In reading cancer literature I was aware that sleep was an opportunity to strengthen my body's natural powers to regenerate my cells and push back against cancer. My sleeplessness persisted despite counter fights by practising head yoga, using relaxation methods, night time warm baths, herbal teas, warm drinks consisting of turmeric and saffron, listening to soft music, devotional recitations and taking melatonin. My desperation for sleep was exacerbated with the knowledge that sleep was essential to my body's cellular health, repairing damaged cells and strengthening my immune system. Having been a teacher and head of a department in a college, I had never engaged in shift-work and could not understand my challenges with sleep.

Could my problem be the cause of extreme distress due to stress? Was stress truly responsible for my plight? I have a loving husband, three wonderful children with adorable grandkids that I am devoted to, successful careers and after decades of hard work and following rules set by governments, academic institutions and other people, I was finally at a point when I could live the way I wanted and now I had a major unexpected hurdle to overcome. Why should I not be stressed? Stress obviously was a contributor!

Managing two to three hours of sleep on prescribed sleeping pills provided a poor solution as I felt like a zombie, feeling ill-rested and hallucinating on account of these sleeping tablets. I was a chronic insomniac and my oncologist changed my prescription for sleep three to four times but to no avail as none gave me the quality of sleep I craved. My desperation for a good night's rest was accompanied by a host of other troubling ailments. Chemotherapy drugs were killing cancer cells but in the process resulted in a bitter palate and my inability to taste and eat. In addition to my peeling nails which caused painful cracks and bleedings fingers, other side effects were skin discoloration to ash grey, nose bleeds, excessive pain in the joints and inability to read due to watering eyes. I have never considered television to be an entertaining medium and in my state of fragility and brain fog I rejected it entirely. A serious case of brain fog had taken home and accomplishing the smallest of tasks seemed insurmountable. As a once-successful career woman, I was now relegated to an inability to think quickly, remember things and sometimes even hold a conversation. I lost my powers of concentration to cloudiness, lethargy, lack of energy or enthusiasm for anything, including my passion for gardening. For the first time in my adult life I had planted nothing! I felt like a mouse trapped in a hole and could not find its way out. My vivid recollection of those dark moments of emptiness, confusion and state of not being myself were troubling. I was hospitalized thrice due to chemotherapy effects. I now ask myself a simple question as to how I coped to overcome that dreadful time of my life?

Without the slightest hesitation I know it was hope coupled with a supportive family, friends and Regina's community support groups. I can't imagine coping with my difficult time without my husband and soul-mate Zahir, who was my pillar of support physically, emotionally, and mentally. He was my care provider, motivator 24/7, encouraging me to enjoy my environment by taking me for short walks, driving me to parks to enjoy the fresh air, taking me to farmer's market, constantly reminding me of our future plans and the many blessings we had been bestowed with and shared. In his kind consideration he took to learning how to cook to relieve me of this responsibility. What more could I have asked for or been blessed with? But there were more caring angels who cared for my well-being.

None of my children lived in Regina but Zahir's brother and wife did (my sister and brother-in-law) and were priceless in the emotional, physical and mental strength they provided especially in my initial months of treatment. They were of invaluable moral support for Zahir who needed the strength as the sole care provider. My sister-in-law, being a physician, extended compassion, empathy, and proved to be an essential resource in sorting many challenges and varied issues that arose. Our children demonstrated their immense affection and concern through regular contact via social mediums. My daughter and her husband lived in Jordan with their three kids under six years of age. Despite our shrinking world and ease of air travel, it would take forty-eight hours of air travel to Regina. My two sons, living in Toronto and Saskatoon, were frequent visitors which was heart-warming, and a great source of encouragement and caring. Consistent communication of all loved ones provided additional crucial motivation to fight the disease.

The brutality of knowing you have cancer and its treatment through chemotherapy requires toughness, determination, hope and help. Concerns, prayers, sharing stories and knowledge of well-wishers gave me the inner strength and courage to battle my way forward. One of my most helpful coping mechanisms was sharing my cancer issues with friends, acquaintances and other afflicted individuals fighting their battle against cancer. Although every journey is unique there are many similar coping mechanisms and issues of relevance that I was able to incorporate to help me in my personal journey and sort myself out of this mess.

Life adds more meaning and becomes better appreciated after a gruelling fight with cancer. Father's Day coincided with our wedding anniversary and our children on the pretext of celebrating Father's day planned a 45th wedding anniversary party. My eldest son and his wife had pre-informed us of their travel plans to celebrate Father's day with us. My overwhelming pleasure and surprise to meet my daughter and my sons and daughter-in-law not only for Father's day but a surprise anniversary party was mind-blowing. The party was hosted at Hotel Saskatchewan, a CN hotel maintaining its historic charm, sophistication and grandeur, providing a perfect location to celebrate our anniversary, Father's Day, family reunion and my mid-point in road to recovery. Many of our friends in Regina and its proximity attended and unanimously enjoyed the enticing Prairie cuisine. I could not believe celebrating 45 years of marriage as the years have passed so swiftly and the celebration exceeded our expectations. The whole experience is one of the happiest memories of my life which I will treasure. The timing for this celebration coincided with a bleak moment in my path to recovery and could not have been better timed in cheering me out of my feelings of being entrapped.

The cancer support groups in Regina were fantastic and I tried to take full advantage of the group meetings and activities. The Bodhi Tree Yoga offered a couple of free exclusive yoga classes for breast cancer and other cancer patients. I attended both sessions and got to know the owner/instructor who was a remarkably kind and positive individual. New friendships were kindled either because of a similar predicament to myself or had overcome the worst phase of their journey. The positive energy in the class proved to be a magnetic draw prompting me to look forward to these classes. A cancer survivor psychologist, organized bimonthly get-togethers at her home over cookies and herbal teas to discuss personal issues, anxieties and concerns. Discussions were useful in resolving my personal demons and helped me understand that I was not alone in my journey of suffering. It taught me that there is life after cancer and I must not let the disease define me.

The greatest impact and source of enjoyment I experienced was from an art and meditation therapy class I attended for eight weeks funded by the Saskatchewan Arts Board. I was on a steep learning curve in these classes. The instructor, Bonnie Chapman, drew co-relations between art forms, symbolisms and skillfully mashed meditation and meditative reflections to different art forms and mediums. She successfully created a peaceful, serene and meaningful environment enabling creativity to flow. These classes touched my inner core releasing my anxieties, fears and apprehensions. From feeling like a mouse trapped in a hole I was psychologically crawling out challenging my mischievous monkey mind to move away allowing me to feel calm, safe and secure as an elephant. I coined my final art piece, Mandala (captioned below), and upon its completion I could see the periphery of the art depicting dark clouds and stormy seas upon which I was floating. There is a rainbow on the side and a face surrounded by light in the center looking out at the world. I understood this face to be mine looking to embrace the world. I finally felt freedom, love, laughter and tranquility through this art. I learnt that capturing quality of life was up to me. My classes were engaging and relaxing to the point that Zahir informed my instructor that "Roshan is smiling when she comes out of these sessions." Affliction with cancer had inflicted me with a darkness where I had forgotten to smile, laugh or show any emotion and these classes enabled me to heal, grow and evolve.

Incredulously, creative art had offered me a lifeline helping my vulnerability. Rumi's quote 'don't get lost in your pain and know that one day your pain will become your cure' resonates deeply as my painting was the beginning of my recovery. Creative art was both a source of inspiration and consolation giving me strength to test the boundaries of art. I have often been asked to describe the process of change. I am challenged to describe this emotional change but can ascribe to this art bringing hope at a time of hopelessness and when I was weak it gave me strength to a sense of well-being and I was able to break out in a smile.

It allowed me a different perspective with a snapshot of my situation. I suddenly was able to interpret, analyze and understand my complex situation as full of versatility and multiplicity of answers. Its very diversity was fascinating and my thinking was brought to focus and clarity, allowing me to relax and smile. I fully appreciated that my piece of art could be what I wanted it to be.

Ray of Hope

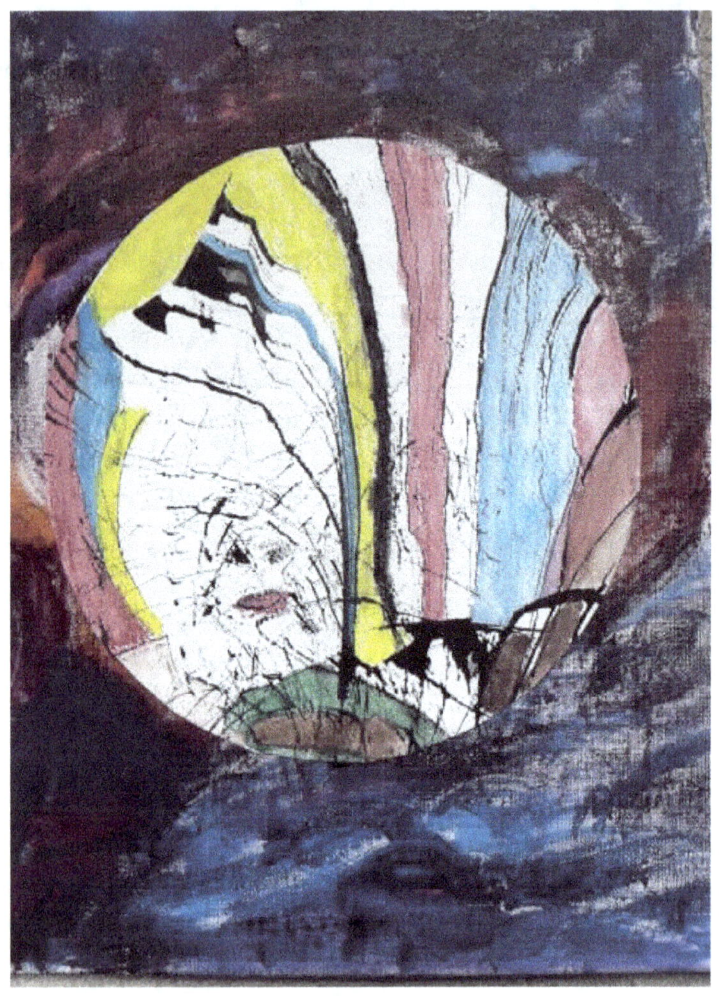

Mandala by Roshan Hemani

Cancer is horrific and I have a new appreciation for how devastating and unpredictable this fatal disease can be. I eventually recognized that my treatment had played havoc with my mind, cluttering it with messy thoughts. I realized that time would give me the strength and courage to resume quality life after my current dark phase. Gradually, I regained my confidence with a shift of the mind and heart and became stronger physically, mentally and emotionally. I was walking three miles every morning with Zahir and started to enjoy nature.

I would like to share an example of a friend's journey with cancer that helped me strengthen my fight. The same time when I was going through my diagnosis and treatment I learnt of a friend who was battling stage four lung cancer and had been given six months of life in the professional opinion of her oncologist. The devastating news prompted her family and friends to commence a 40 day vigil of prayers and devotional hymns for her, myself and others afflicted with cancer.

To the surprise of the medical staff, seven years later, despite their grim prediction, my friend is alive. At the time, I too was at a critical period traveling through unpredictability of the effects of this disease. Despite my fragile condition I participated with faith, conviction and hope in these prayers. My habitual recitation of devotional hymns prior to bedtime gave me remarkable spiritual strength and resolve to fight this sinister disease. I have spent the past seven wonderful years indulging every wish in my bucket list including giving back unconditionally, gardening, helping humanity, travelling to exotic destinations, making more friends and fulfilling a satisfying spiritual life.

Upon much reflection, I deemed it essential to share lessons learnt through my journey as an effective medium for providing encouragement to those wrestling with similar or comparable health issues.

1. Hang on tight to your faith and prayers, no matter how much your mind wanders, learn to ignore your loss of focus. Praying with conviction provides inner strength and hope.

2. My narrative of the path to recovery may resonate with you and enable you to deploy some of the techniques shared. Where there is hope, there is the inner motivation to take baby steps towards recovery and feeling better. Every step is important as it converts liability into assets and keeps despondency at bay. Talk about your cancer freely as there is no reason to hide or lie as it is a pretentious mask to be shed. Accept your condition and deal with it from the onset.

3. Explore different avenues of support in your community. It cultivates bonds of solidarity and you may forge friendships with others who are trying to balance their lives. Give support groups time and stay with the ones that resonate with you.

4. Maintain contact with your friends and acquaintances where energy permits. Enjoy your natural environment and expose yourself to moments of pleasure from visit to farmers markets, shows, museums etc. These are great distractions and provide fun and laughter.

5. It is easy to become self centered as you become accustomed to attention. The most precious person is your significant other and your care provider. He/she is also on an emotional roller coaster and it

is essential that you are sensitive to their feelings and needs.

6. I understand it takes five years to clear cancer drugs from your system and I was further prescribed Letrozole to be taken for five more years after to decrease my chances of recurrence. After careful evaluation of its risks and benefits, I opted not to take the additional drug because of its side effects. You have a choice, so make informed decisions.

Life as a cancer survivor has brought many blessings for which I am deeply grateful. I excitedly returned to Arusha, Tanzania. Completing the project I had initially been assigned brought the greatest satisfaction, inner happiness, contentment and serenity. I planted 160,000 trees on the site and working close to nature proved highly therapeutic. I am full of gratitude to the Divine for eradicating the worst phase of my life to one that is rich with wisdom and tolerance and has more depth than ever before as I treat life and its resources with utmost respect.

When Naila requested me to share my personal journey and experience with cancer I was in immediate agreement for many reasons. I strongly believe in sharing lessons learnt with others coupled with my admiration, love and respect for Naila who too has been valiantly and courageously battling her cancer. My fervent prayers and best wishes to Naila, Shamshad, and others afflicted, to find inner strength and balance to navigate through this phase of life for *it too shall pass.*

About the author

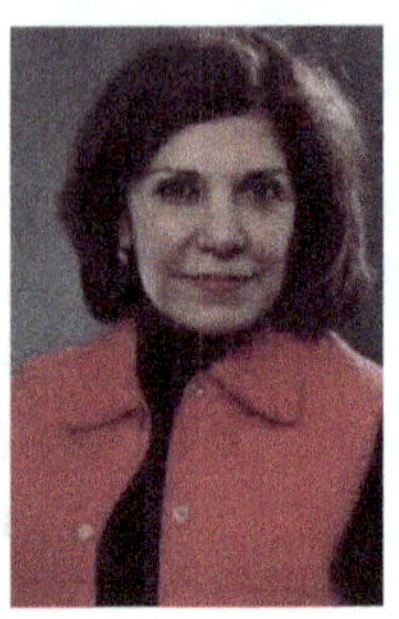

Naila Abdulla enjoys over 25 years' experience in the tourism sector with academic credentials from respected Universities: Harvard, George Washington University and a PhD in tourism development from the University of Waterloo. She has travelled through 44 countries and has experience with tourism development in the Bahamas, Cuba, Caribbean, Mexico, Florida and Kenya. Business and academic acumen uniquely position Dr. Abdulla to volunteer her retirement years to integrate business with development for sustainable programs for diverse cultures, environmental impacts and skill transfers for an improved labor pool. She is retired and lives in Calgary, Alberta.

FIGHT CANCER is a true narrative of how morbid cancer has dominated my life in a pervasive manner from changing my vocabulary to almost daily treatment visits. Every cancer narrative hums inspiring tales of being courageous with anecdotal capture of pain, suffering, endurance, courage, hope and fight because that is a true depiction of a cancer patient's life. How can any story be different? Fear of cancer is linked to mortality and a wake-up call for being on borrowed time. The outstanding group of focused and disciplined stakeholders come equipped with kindness, compassion, programs, services, new treatments and therapies, **but they cannot make it go away**.

My family history has been at war against aggressive cancer and I have lost several cousins, aunts, uncles including my mother 50 years ago and sister 25 years ago after a fight with this demonic disease…... I ask, are we any further ahead to 50 years ago? **The fight I speak of is not only to fight the disease but to fight for a cure.** I am not a professional writer nor interested in earning a profit from this book as nominal proceeds generated will go to Tom Baker Cancer Centre. I have an eagerness to convey that life is bigger than cancer and though **humanitarian causes do not get as much ink or respect as profit making enterprises you are not alone**. If I as a single woman, living alone, in a new province, city and neighbourhood can make it, so can you!

I hope this short read will create an awareness and resonate with you. I am a private person publicly sharing my journey in the hope that I can inspire your fight. Medical insights are a task beyond my competence but this personal narrative details various processes, what I learnt, what you should know, how to cope and manage with your situation, programs and services available and suggestions to strengthen your spirit.

References:

https://www.bing.com/search?q=breast+cancer+deaths+worldwide&form=EDGEAR&qs=PF&cvid=fc152ecc2) Retrieved March 17, 2020

https://www.canada.ca/.../chronic-diseases/cancer/breast-cancer Retrieved March 17, 2020

https://www.breastcancer.org/symptoms/diagnosis/brca Retrieved March 18, 2020

https://www.nationalbreastcancer.org/breast-cancer-risk-factors Retrieved March 18, 2020.

https://www.ctvnews.ca/health/cancer-cases-expected-to-soar-40-per-cent-by-2030 Retrieved March 21, 2020

https://www.cancer.gov/about-cancer/understanding/what-is-cancer Retrieved March 23, 2020

https://www.cancer.ca/~/media/cancer.ca/CW/publications/Canadian%20Cancer%20Statistics/Canadian-Cancer-Statistics-2019-EN.pdf Retrieved April 20,2020

https://www.ama-assn.org/delivering-care/precision-medicine/genetic-testing Retrieved 23 March, 2020.

https://www.cancer.gov/about-cancer/causes-prevention/genetics/genetic-testing-fact-sheet Retrieved March 23, 2020

https://www.forbes.com/sites/quora/2018/09/10/some-think-big-pharma-is...Retrieved on April 27, 2020 https://www.healthline.com/health/triple-negative-breast-cancer-recurrence Retrieved April 29, 2020

https://www.cancer.ca/~/media/cancer.ca/CW/publications /Breast%20cancer%20UYD/32064-1-NO.pdf Retrieved on April 20,2020

https://www.soas.ac.uk/cedep-demos/000_P500_ESM_K3736-Demo/unit1/page_08.htm Retrieved April 20, 20

https://www.searchquotes.com/quotes/about/Life_Lesson/ #ixzz6LJ9W18Ra Retrieved on April 29,2020

Text taken from Dr. Paul Leon Masters' Book, "Mystical Insights: Knowing the Unknown," Pgs. 42–45. Copyright © 2016 by the International Metaphysical Ministry.

Waajiman, Kees (2002) Spirituality: Forms, Foundations, methods, Peeters Publishers. <u>Waaijman 2002</u>, p. 315

The Cancer Sleeper Cell. A version of this article appears in print on Oct. 31, 2010, page 40, of the Sunday Magazine. Siddhartha Mukherjee is an assistant professor of medicine in the division of medical oncology at Columbia University. This article is adapted from his book "Emperor of All Maladies: A Biography of Cancer,"

www.ingramcontent.com/pod-product-compliance
Lightning Source LLC
Chambersburg PA
CBHW061005050726
47592CB00003B/1359